# *Delavier's* Mixed Martial Arts Anatomy

## Frédéric Delavier
## Michael Gundill

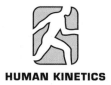

**HUMAN KINETICS**

**PART 3**

# TRAINING PROGRAMS 126

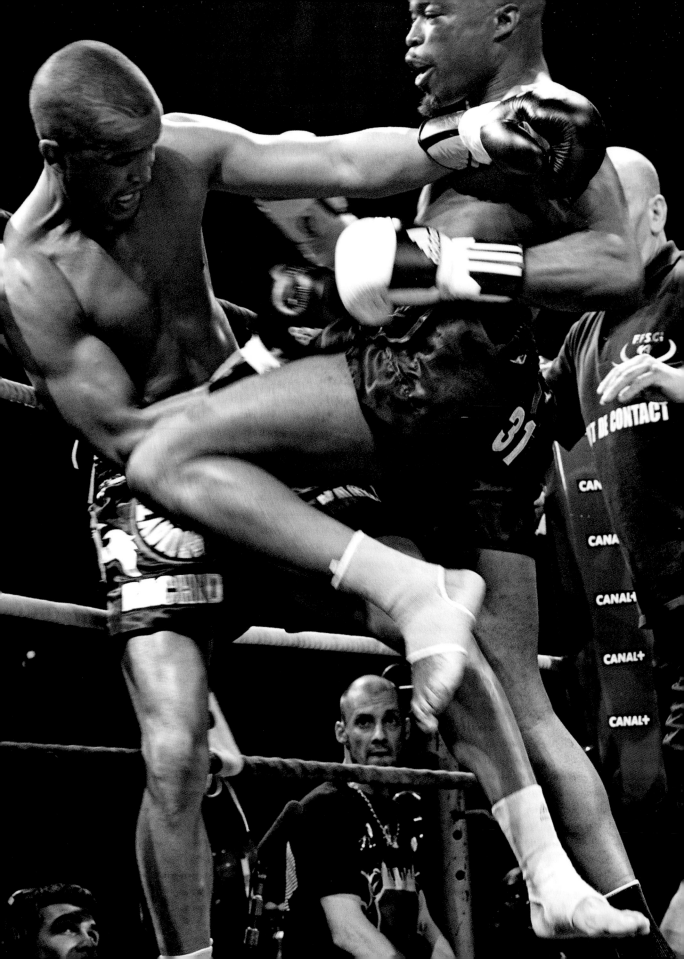

# WHY YOU SHOULD STRENGTH TRAIN

Strength training has become indispensable for mixed martial arts because it improves your effectiveness in five ways:

❶ It makes your strikes more powerful.

❷ It develops endurance and resistance.

❸ It increases the range of motion in your movements (for example, in your kicks).

❹ It creates a protective armor that reduces your vulnerability in a fight.

❺ It prevents overuse injuries. The repetitive nature of violent strikes can cause premature damage to muscles and joints. Strength training helps prevent this trauma so that you can avoid unnecessary injuries.

## THE KEY IS EFFECTIVENESS

No fighter has hours and hours to devote to strength training. Since your ability to recover is limited, the time you devote to strength training must, to some degree, be taken away from the time you spend practicing fighting techniques.

You should focus your strength training program on the essentials in the following ways:

❶ Focus exclusively on what works best. We show you that certain exercises, even though they are very popular, are a waste of time since they do not correspond well with the neuromuscular effort required in a fight.

❷ Tailor your training program to your specific needs as precisely as possible.

We focus on these two points throughout this book so that you will achieve maximum results in the shortest time.

## OUR GOAL IS SIMPLICITY

An infinite number of accessories and gadgets are available for strength training and martial arts. If we ignore what is fashionable at the moment, we see that most of these tools are far from necessary. In reality, a weight bar and dumbbells are more than sufficient for excellent strength training. We have designed the core of our programs around these two instruments, since everyone has access to them and they are, by far, the most effective.

## USING THE ANATOMOMORPHOLOGICAL APPROACH TO FIGHTING IN YOUR STRENGTH TRAINING

In the past, fighting techniques taught as part of a discipline had very little chance of being appropriate for an individual's morphology (body type). The major revolution in free fighting is that you can select the techniques that are best suited to your own morphology.

You will adapt this philosophy to strength training so you can avoid the mistake of copying what a friend or what a champion fighter does. Everyone has a unique morphology, and to be the best fighter you can be, you must respect these physiological requirements. Therefore, we explain how to adapt strength training exercises to your morphology.

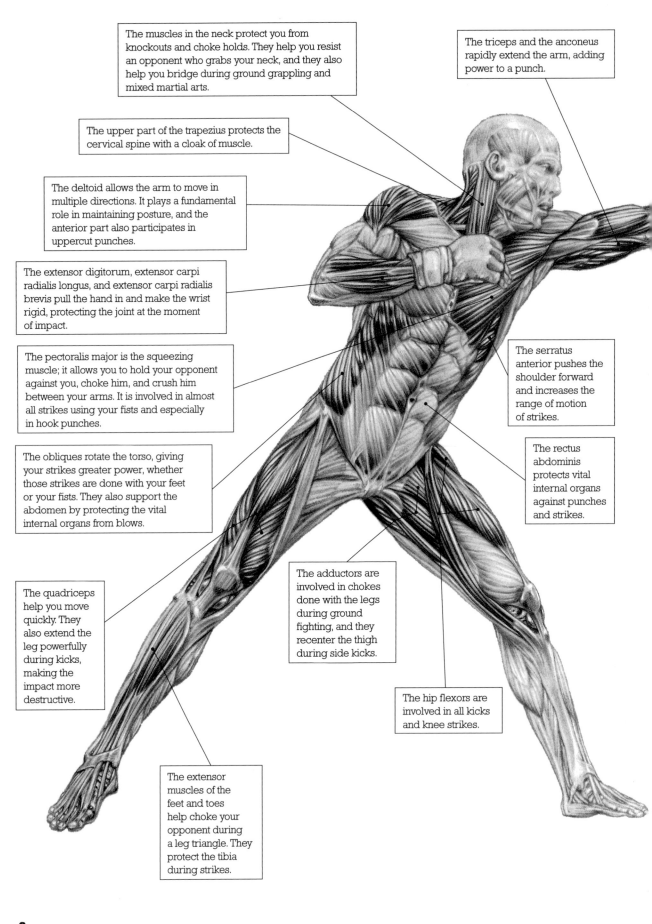

The muscles in the neck protect you from knockouts and choke holds. They help you resist an opponent who grabs your neck, and they also help you bridge during ground grappling and mixed martial arts.

The triceps and the anconeus rapidly extend the arm, adding power to a punch.

The upper part of the trapezius protects the cervical spine with a cloak of muscle.

The deltoid allows the arm to move in multiple directions. It plays a fundamental role in maintaining posture, and the anterior part also participates in uppercut punches.

The extensor digitorum, extensor carpi radialis longus, and extensor carpi radialis brevis pull the hand in and make the wrist rigid, protecting the joint at the moment of impact.

The serratus anterior pushes the shoulder forward and increases the range of motion of strikes.

The pectoralis major is the squeezing muscle; it allows you to hold your opponent against you, choke him, and crush him between your arms. It is involved in almost all strikes using your fists and especially in hook punches.

The rectus abdominis protects vital internal organs against punches and strikes.

The obliques rotate the torso, giving your strikes greater power, whether those strikes are done with your feet or your fists. They also support the abdomen by protecting the vital internal organs from blows.

The adductors are involved in chokes done with the legs during ground fighting, and they recenter the thigh during side kicks.

The quadriceps help you move quickly. They also extend the leg powerfully during kicks, making the impact more destructive.

The hip flexors are involved in all kicks and knee strikes.

The extensor muscles of the feet and toes help choke your opponent during a leg triangle. They protect the tibia during strikes.

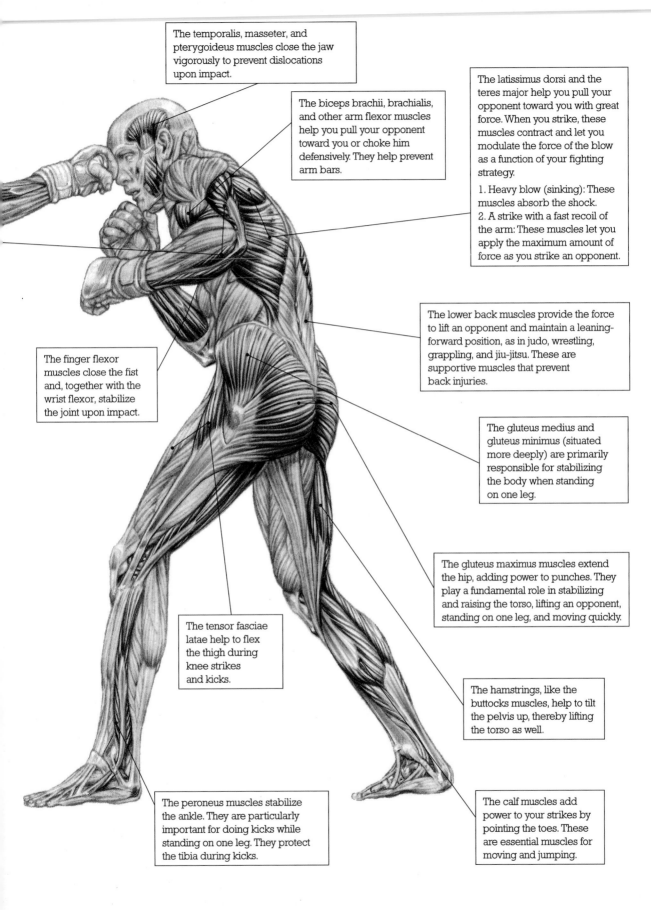

The temporalis, masseter, and pterygoideus muscles close the jaw vigorously to prevent dislocations upon impact.

The biceps brachii, brachialis, and other arm flexor muscles help you pull your opponent toward you or choke him defensively. They help prevent arm bars.

The latissimus dorsi and the teres major help you pull your opponent toward you with great force. When you strike, these muscles contract and let you modulate the force of the blow as a function of your fighting strategy.

1. Heavy blow (sinking): These muscles absorb the shock.
2. A strike with a fast recoil of the arm: These muscles let you apply the maximum amount of force as you strike an opponent.

The lower back muscles provide the force to lift an opponent and maintain a leaning-forward position, as in judo, wrestling, grappling, and jiu-jitsu. These are supportive muscles that prevent back injuries.

The finger flexor muscles close the fist and, together with the wrist flexor, stabilize the joint upon impact.

The gluteus medius and gluteus minimus (situated more deeply) are primarily responsible for stabilizing the body when standing on one leg.

The gluteus maximus muscles extend the hip, adding power to punches. They play a fundamental role in stabilizing and raising the torso, lifting an opponent, standing on one leg, and moving quickly.

The tensor fasciae latae help to flex the thigh during knee strikes and kicks.

The hamstrings, like the buttocks muscles, help to tilt the pelvis up, thereby lifting the torso as well.

The peroneus muscles stabilize the ankle. They are particularly important for doing kicks while standing on one leg. They protect the tibia during kicks.

The calf muscles add power to your strikes by pointing the toes. These are essential muscles for moving and jumping.

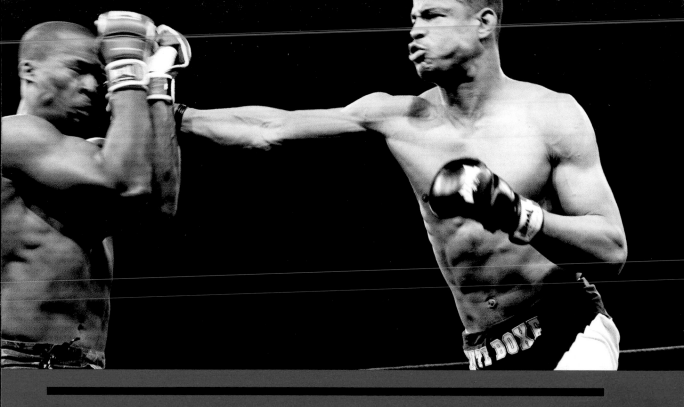

# PRINCIPLES OF
# STRENGTH TRAINING

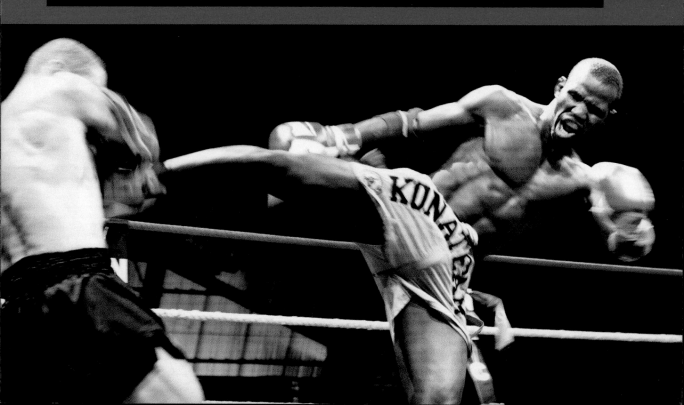

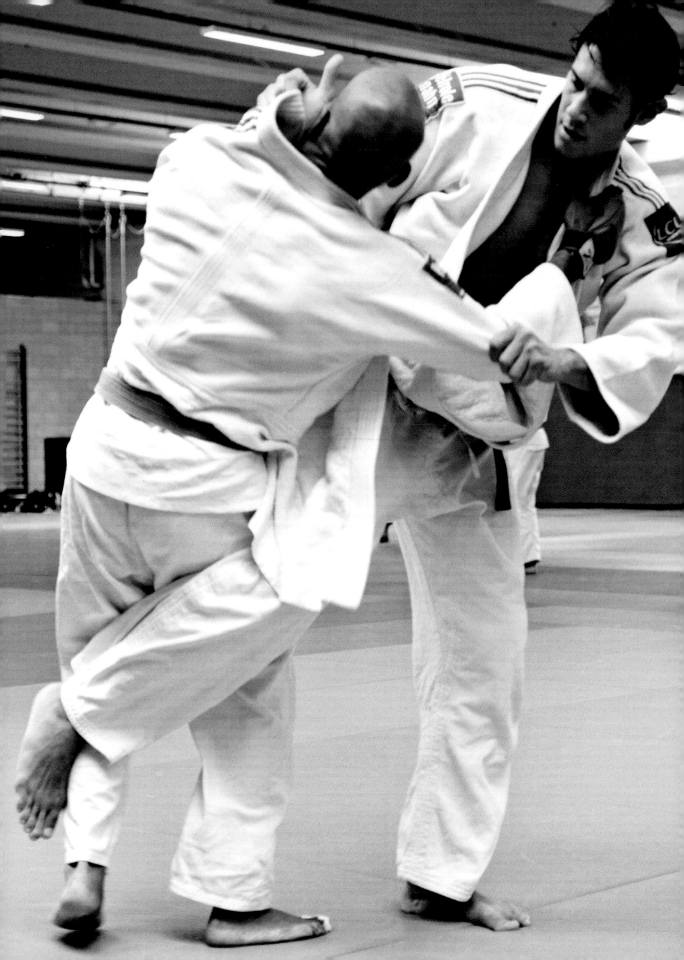

# DEVELOPING YOUR PROGRAM

## 20 STEPS TO DEVELOPING YOUR TRAINING PROGRAM

To develop a customized weight training program, we rely on basic theory that is very important to understand. Proceeding methodically, we describe each of the 20 steps that are the key to your personalized program. Once you have gone through these 20 steps, you will have answered all the questions about developing your strength training program.

### 1 Define Your Goals

The first step in creating a strength training program is to clearly define your goals.

Do you want to do any of the following?

→ Get stronger
→ Improve power
→ Strengthen specific areas
→ Increase the effectiveness of certain strikes
→ Increase your cardiorespiratory fitness
→ Strengthen your whole body

Often, you have multiple goals in mind. But if you do not clearly define those goals, it will be difficult to create an optimal program, because particular training techniques correspond to each of your goals.

Then, you must quantify your goals. For example, would you like to do any of the following?

→ Lift 10 pounds (about 5 kg) more with your arms in 1 month

→ Double the number of sets you can do in 10 minutes so that you can increase your endurance in 15 days
→ Increase the size of your neck by half an inch in 2 months

The time frame and the rate of progress that you set must be realistic. Keep in mind that no one reaches goals as quickly as desired! More often than not, people feel they have hit a plateau. However, with a good program, true plateaus are rare. If you define your goals and establish regular and precise steps to reach along the way, you will be able to measure your progress easily. Every time you achieve a step, you will be motivated to keep training.

Standard programs are provided in part 3 (page 126). These are basic programs that you can customize according to various parameters that we will discuss.

### 2 How Many Times Should You Train Each Week?

Your schedule is the determining factor in answering this question. Unfortunately, your schedule does not always permit you the optimal amount of time. But know that even if you can strength train only once a week, it is still better than not exercising at all. You will still make progress. If you are a beginning fighter who already trains intensely for fights, one strength training session per week should suffice.

However, we think that two weight training sessions per week are appropriate. Three workouts a week should be more than enough, unless you want to suffer a large loss of strength. We recommend that you not go beyond four workouts a week. Overtraining is more damaging to your progress than undertraining. Only excellent athletes will benefit from more than four sessions per week.

### ⚠ WARNING!

When you start strength training, you are generally full of enthusiasm and energy. You feel like working out every day so you can make a lot of progress.

This much enthusiasm at the beginning could turn into disillusionment as well as fatigue (overtraining), and then you could lose motivation. Fighters who know how to ration efforts will get the most benefit from strength training. Results do not happen instantly, so you must be patient.

### ♦ EVOLUTION

Ideally, you should start with one or two weekly sessions for a month or two before moving to three sessions when you feel ready. At first, do not work out more than three times per week. After three to six months of regular training, you could plan out a four-day program.

### ❸ On Which Days Should You Exercise?

Ideally, you should alternate one day of weight training with one day of rest. But again, this might not fit your schedule. In that case, you have to find a balance between the ideal and your own abilities.

Following are options for programs:

### ♦ ONE WORKOUT PER WEEK

You can choose any day you like.

### ♦ TWO WORKOUTS PER WEEK

Weight training sessions should be spaced out as far as possible. An example is Monday and Thursday or Tuesday and Friday. In any case, give yourself at least one day of rest between two workouts. The exception, of course, is if you are able to work out only on the weekends. Strength training for two consecutive days is not ideal, but you will have the rest of the week to recover.

### ♦ THREE WORKOUTS PER WEEK

The best plan is to alternate a day of training with a day of rest. For example, work out on Monday, Wednesday, and Friday. This way your whole weekend is free. It is still possible to do strength training on two consecutive days (on the weekend, for example) and do the third workout on Wednesday, but you should avoid this if possible. The worst program would have you training three days in a row. The only way to justify this is if your schedule absolutely requires it.

### ♦ FOUR WORKOUTS PER WEEK

For this schedule, you have the fewest rest days and therefore you will have to work out two days in a row.

Here are examples:

→ Monday, Wednesday, Friday, Sunday
→ Monday, Tuesday, Thursday, Saturday

If your schedule is flexible, you could spread these four training sessions out over eight days instead of seven. This way, one day of training will always be followed by one day of rest. Recovery will be optimized due to the slightly longer training intervals. The only drawback is that your workout days will change from week to week on this program.

## ⚠ WARNING!

Knowing how many times you should strength train each week comes back to knowing how many rest days to give yourself between two workouts.

Muscles grow stronger during the rest period between two workouts and not during the actual workout. So it is just as important to rest as it is to exercise.

If you are not getting stronger or gaining more endurance from one workout to the next, it would be wise to give your muscles more time to recover. Lack of progress is a sure sign that you are not getting enough rest.

## ④ How Many Muscles Should You Work in Each Session?

To answer this question, you need to know the distinction between training for muscle mass (bodybuilding) and training to improve fighting skills. A bodybuilder isolates each muscle group as much as possible. For example, a bodybuilder works the upper body one day and works the lower body on a different day.

Following this artificial segmentation is a serious mistake for a fighter. To make progress as a fighter, you need to train all the muscles on the same day because, in a fight, these muscles work together, not separately.

The only exception is if you need to focus specifically on one part of the body (neck or abdomen, for example).

## ⑤ Should You Work Your Muscles in a Particular Order?

The body is made up of six large body regions (see the illustrations on the next page):

→ Arms (biceps, triceps, forearms)
→ Back (neck, trapezius, latissimus dorsi, lumbar region)
→ Shoulders
→ Chest
→ Abdomen
→ Thighs and lower legs (quadriceps, hamstrings, buttocks, shins, and calves)

There are dozens of possible combinations for working these six large body regions, but they are not all good. This is why we explain how to reduce the number of possibilities so that you can focus on the most effective combinations.

The proper order for working your muscles depends on these aspects:

→ Some commonsense rules you should follow
→ The priority you have given each group
→ Your flexibility as a function of your progress

♦ 1. THE RULES
A few rules apply to most fighters:

→ Do not work your arms before your chest, shoulders, or back. For the latter three groups, you will need the strength in your arms. Your arm muscles must not be too tired when you begin working your torso muscles.
→ For your legs, you should always work the calves last. When your calves are tired, they might begin to shake when you really push the thighs. This shaking not only will decrease your performance, but it could also be dangerous (you could fall).

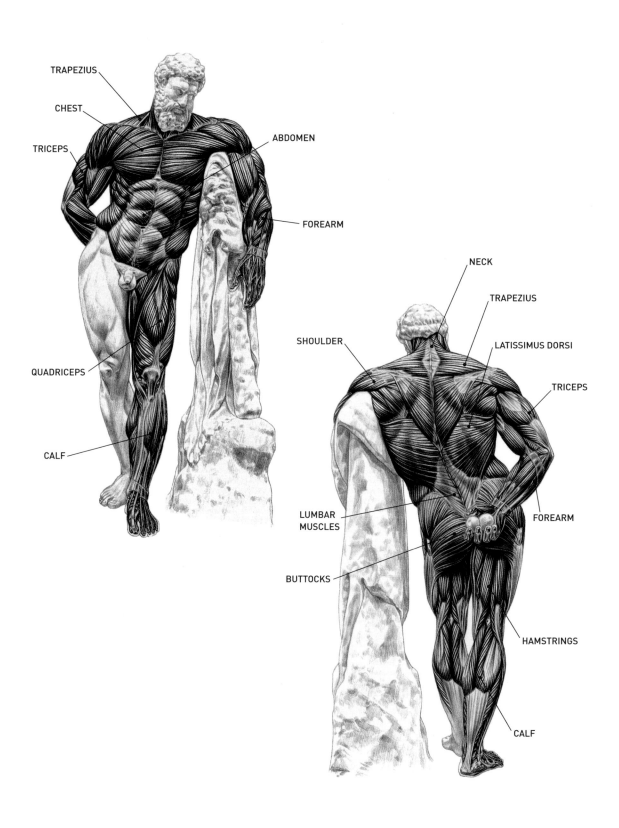

TRAPEZIUS

CHEST

TRICEPS

ABDOMEN

FOREARM

QUADRICEPS

CALF

NECK

TRAPEZIUS

SHOULDER

LATISSIMUS DORSI

TRICEPS

FOREARM

LUMBAR
MUSCLES

BUTTOCKS

HAMSTRINGS

CALF

→ Alternate one exercise for the upper body with one for the lower body. Then go back to the upper body and so on. For example, work the chest, quadriceps, shoulders, hamstrings, and back. So while the upper body is recovering, the lower body is working. This will allow you to lift heavier weights.

### ♦ 2. YOUR PRIORITIES

The second item that will determine the order in which you work your muscles is your priorities. So, all muscles will not necessarily be treated the same way.

Your priorities should dictate the structure of your training program. You must keep in mind that when you focus on certain muscles, other muscles will be neglected a bit since your workout capacity is limited.

As a fighter, you should rank the importance of each muscle group according to your fighting style. As an example, for a boxer, the shoulders, arms, and abdomen are particularly important.

For a kickboxer, the focus is on the thighs rather than the upper back. Focusing on the muscles of the upper body while letting the thighs go a little bit means the muscles in the torso will progress at a faster rate and vice versa.

If you have a weak spot (the abdomen, for example), you can begin your workouts with abdominal exercises as a kind of warm-up. However, a strong area or a muscle that is not critical to your fighting style could be left until the end of a session. You can work that area more or less intensely depending on your energy level and how much time you have left to work out.

### ♦ 3. FLEXIBILITY AS A FUNCTION OF YOUR PROGRESS

You must realize that your priorities are not set in stone. They constantly evolve. The more progress you make, the more you have to adjust your program to adapt to the new environment. For example, compared to an experienced fighter, the strength of a beginner's punch comes from the following areas (Filimonov et al, 1985, *NSCA Journal*, 7(6), 65-66):

→ 38% from the arm (versus 25% for a champion boxer)

→ 45% from the rotation of the torso (37% for a champion)

→ 17% from the back leg (38% for a champion)

So, to improve your punches as a beginner, you do not need to work the thighs as much as a champion does. In this way, you can avoid wasting time on your legs when you should focus on the arms and torso rotation. Physical preparation should adapt to the fighting style, not the other way around.

The better you become as a fighter, the more the force of your punch will come from your thighs, which suggests that the importance given to various muscles will change as you progress. You will have to modify your strength training program over time.

## 6 How Many Sets of Each Exercise Should You Do?

**DEFINITION**

A set is the number of repetitions of the same exercise until you reach fatigue.

The number of sets per exercise is an important factor in your progress. If you do too many sets, you will overtrain, and that will limit your progress. If you do not do enough sets, the muscles will not be stimulated optimally to achieve quick results.

Your experience level determines the approximate number of sets that you should do for each exercise.

★ **Beginners:** Do no more than three sets per exercise.
★ **After one month of training:** Do no more than four sets per exercise.
★ **After two months of training:** Do no more than five sets per exercise.
★ **After three months of training:** Do no more than six sets per exercise.
★ **Beyond three months:** You will be able to determine the number of sets as a function of your needs as well as your ability to recover.

## ⚠ WARNING!

The goal is not to do a bunch of easy sets so you can reach a magic number. It is better to push yourself during every set and end up doing fewer total sets than the alternative. If you have no difficulty going beyond these maximum limits, it means the intensity of your muscle contraction is not high enough. This intensity comes with time as you train. Your muscles cannot push beyond their physical possibilities during a set from one day to the next.

### Note
Since warm-up sets are less intense, you should not include these sets in your total set count.

## HOW TO ADJUST YOUR WORKOUT VOLUME

The number of sets is the first variable you can change when you adjust your workout volume. Changing the number of sets allows you to make smaller adjustments than just adding exercises, but you will have to play around with it at first. As you become stronger, and when you feel ready, add a set here and there.

The best thing is to let your muscles tell you how many sets you should do. The most obvious indicator is when you start to lose strength abnormally from one set to the next. An abrupt loss of strength means you have probably done one too many sets.

Obviously, the number of sets that you can do might fluctuate from one workout to the next. On days when you are feeling great, you might be tempted to add sets. But on days when you are feeling tired, go ahead and reduce the number of sets so that you do not exhaust yourself.

## 7 How Many Sets Should You Do in Each Workout?

Your fitness level, schedule, and goals will determine the total number of sets that you can do during a workout.

♦ **BASIC GUIDELINES FOR CLASSIC STRENGTH TRAINING**
★ **Beginners:** Do no more than 10 sets per workout.
★ **After one month of training:** Do no more than 12 sets per workout.
★ **After two months of training:** Do no more than 15 sets per workout.
★ **After three months of training:** Do no more than 20 sets per workout.

♦ **BASIC GUIDELINES FOR CONDITIONING**
★ **Beginners:** Do no more than 12 sets per workout.
★ **After one month of training:** Do no more than 15 sets per workout.
★ **After two months of training:** Do no more than 20 sets per workout.
★ **After three months of training:** Do no more than 25 sets per workout.

## ❽ When Should You Change Exercises?

As your muscles grow, you must constantly adjust your workout program. Beginners make rapid progress, especially when doing the same workout week after week. As long as your routine is producing results, it makes perfect sense to keep doing it. Changing the structure too often creates negative interference, slowing down motor learning and preventing a gradual increase in the intensity of the workout.

Basically, muscles cannot give their best effort on a new exercise. They require an initiation period (called motor learning) to be able to mobilize all their strength. This is why you make rapid progress on a new exercise over several workouts: You started at the bottom, far from your strength potential.

It is difficult for a beginner who is not used to strength training exercises to reach the critical threshold to mobilize strength optimally. If you are a beginner, the best way to increase intensity is to know that you did 10 reps of an exercise during your previous workout and so you need to do at least 11 reps, with good form, today.

If you change your exercises too often, your muscles will not have enough time to learn to work hard during the old exercise. All the time you spend learning a new exercise means less time that you could be getting stronger. Constantly changing exercises when it is not necessary will multiply these nonproductive learning periods.

However, if you notice that your progress has slowed down over several consecutive workouts, then it is time to change your program. The first variable to adjust in a workout program is to change the exercises you are doing.

## ❾ How Many Repetitions Should You Do in a Set?

> **DEFINITION**
>
> The term *repetition* is the total number of times you do an exercise in a set (see the definition of *set* on page 17). A repetition happens in three stages:
> → Positive phase: You use your muscle to lift the weight.
> → Static (isometric) phase: You hold the contracted position.
> → Negative phase: You use your muscle to slow the descent of the weight.

It is normal to wonder how many repetitions you should do during a set. But you should know that there is no magic number that will give you the results you desire. More than repetitions, what really counts is the intensity of the contraction. Adjusting the number of repetitions is just one way to make progress, not an end in and of itself. The best thing to do is to change the number of repetitions as a function of your goals.

★ **Goal: Increase Muscle Mass and Weight**
As a general rule, you will gain muscle mass when you perform 8 to 12 repetitions. But if you can do 13 repetitions at a given weight instead of 12, then do it! But in your next set, you must increase the weight.

★ **Goal: Increase Strength**
To increase your strength, you need to do 3 to 6 repetitions.

★ **Goal: Increase Power**
Power comes from performing explosive (plyometric) exercises in sets of 8 to 10 repetitions.

During plyometric sets, stop the set when the speed of each repetition diminishes noticeably.

★ **Goal: Improve Isometric Endurance**
Isometric, or static, sets include 3 to 6 repetitions. In hand-to-hand combat, the fighter with the best isometric endurance will win.

★ **Goal: Improve Muscular Endurance**
For endurance, you should do circuits with at least 15 repetitions.

## ⑩ How Quickly Should You Perform Repetitions?

♦ **BEGINNING STRENGTH TRAINING PHASE**
To learn to master muscle contraction properly, it is best to start by moving the weight relatively slowly. The worst thing you can do as a beginner is to swing your torso aggressively while twisting and arching your back to lift a weight. This will create bad habits that will be difficult to break. At best, cheating will slow your progress. At worst, you risk injuring yourself! When in doubt, slow the repetition instead of rushing through it.

For heavy work, you should lift the weight using your muscle and without momentum:
→ Take 1 to 2 (true) seconds to lift the weight.
→ Slowly release and take 1 to 2 seconds to lower the weight.

This means a repetition should take 2 to 4 seconds in total. If you go faster, you will not use the full strength of your muscles even if you lift a heavier weight.

♦ **EVOLUTION**
It is imperative that you master basic technique before trying different strategies. As a fighter, once you achieve good muscle control, you can increase the speed of the exercises in order to gain explosiveness.

Explosiveness does not mean cheating. There is a very fine line between plyometric training and losing control. This is why it is important to master the muscle contraction well before moving on to plyometric exercises.

A plyometric repetition is better for the kinds of movements that are required in combat sports. It is very rare for a fighter to move in a slow and controlled manner. Generally, a fighter moves as fast as possible. The goal of plyometric training is to give you this speed.

Once you are familiar with the techniques and have spent a few weeks mastering them, you can adjust the speed of your repetitions to match your goals.

★ **Goal: Increase Muscle Mass and Weight**
You must lift the weight using your muscles and not momentum:
→ Take 2 (true) seconds to lift the weight.
→ Take 2 seconds to lower the weight.

So a repetition should take about 4 seconds in total. If you can do more repetitions by going faster, it means you are using momentum and not the strength of your muscles.

★ **Goal: Increase Strength**

Your repetitions should be accelerated a little bit.

→ Take 1 to 2 seconds to lift the weight (without jerking or twisting).

→ Lower the weight with control, which should take 1 to 2 seconds.

→ As an option: Between repetitions, take a 5- to 10-second break so your muscles can regain their strength (see the between-reps break strategy on page 37).

A repetition should take 2 to 4 seconds in total (not counting rest time between repetitions).

★ **Goal: Increase Power**

The speed of your repetitions increases even more to help you gain explosiveness.

→ Take 1 second to lift the weight.

→ Take 1 second to lower the weight.

→ As an option: Between repetitions, take a 3- to 5-second break so your muscles can regain their strength.

This kind of repetition should take 2 seconds in total (not counting rest time between repetitions).

★ **Goal: Improve Isometric Endurance**

During isometric work, you must push to your maximum. Improved isometric endurance benefits you in the following ways:

→ In an offensive position, it will mean the difference between a quick submission and your opponent getting away.

→ In a defensive position, it will help you break your opponent's hold.

The goal is to hold the contracted position for at least 30 seconds per repetition. When this becomes easy, you need to increase the weight.

★ **Goal: Improve Muscular Endurance**

To increase the number of repetitions you can do, use a little bit of momentum (but do not overdo it). Each repetition will be done dynamically:

→ Lift the weight in less than 1 second.

→ Lower the weight in less than 1 second.

→ Begin the next repetition immediately.

So a single repetition should take less than 2 seconds in total. The muscles stay contracted the entire time. They should never be able to rest. When the burn becomes too intense, take a short break by resting in the relaxed position for a few seconds. Once the lactic acid has dissipated, begin again until the burn becomes intense once more. Take another short break before starting again, and so on.

## ⑪ How Should You Adjust Range of Motion?

You should also adjust the range of motion in your exercises to suit your goals.

★ **Goal: Increase Muscle Mass and Weight**

The range of motion should be as great as possible. Do not overstretch the muscles, or you could suffer an injury.

As you do more sets, if you want to increase the weight you are lifting, you may have to decrease the range of motion at the beginning of the movement.

★ **Goal: Increase Strength**

When you are lifting heavy weights, the lengthening phase is the time you are most susceptible to muscle injury.

As you continue your sets, you can hold the contracted position for a little less time. This will help you do a few more repetitions.

★ **Goal: Increase Power**

The range of motion for each exercise should match the range of motion required in your discipline. Be careful not to overstretch, which can lead to injury.

★ **Goal: Improve Isometric Endurance**

There is no specific range of motion for this goal. Try to match the muscle position as closely as possible to the position you use during a fight when grasping an opponent.

★ **Goal: Improve Muscular Endurance**

To improve endurance in the full length of the muscle, perform the repetitions through a full range of motion.

## ⑫ How Long Should a Workout Last?

The purpose of a good workout is to stimulate the muscles as much as possible in the shortest time. We are careful to favor the intensity of a workout rather than the length.

The first criteria that determine the duration of your workout are your schedule and your availability. If you do not have a lot of time, you should know that it is possible to do a complete workout in a short time (with circuit training, for example). For this, 15 to 20 minutes will suffice (see the conditioning techniques starting on page 41 as well as circuits in the training programs starting on page 135). It is still best to allow at least 30 minutes for a workout.

The length of your workout will depend on two things:

→ Volume of work (number of exercises x number of sets)
→ Rest time between sets

Rest time is the factor you should adjust if you do not have enough time for your workout.

A workout for muscle mass or strength should ideally last for 45 minutes to 1 hour. If you manage to spend more than 1 hour working out, it probably means you were not working out with enough intensity. After 1 hour, your muscles should be begging for mercy.

## ⑬ What Is the Optimal Amount of Rest Between Sets?

Rest time between sets can stretch from just a few seconds to 3 minutes depending on the difficulty of the exercise and your goals.

You need the following:

→ More rest after difficult exercises such as squats and deadlifts
→ Less rest after easier exercises such as those for the neck or the abdominal muscles
→ More rest when you are using heavy weights
→ Less rest when you are using lighter weights

As a general rule, it is time to begin another set if either of the following occurs:

→ When your breathing is almost back to normal
→ When you feel that your enthusiasm is overcoming your fatigue

At first, time yourself so that you stay within the time frame you had set aside for your workout. Timing yourself helps you stay focused. By keeping track of the time, you can better control the intensity and length of your workout.

## ⚠ WARNING!

If your strength decreases abnormally from one set to the next,
→ you might have done too many sets, or
→ you might not have taken enough rest time.
  In the latter case, increase your rest time slightly and see if that solves the problem. If it does not, then inadequate rest time did not cause the decrease in performance, and you did too many sets.

Your goals will determine your rest time more precisely.

★ **Goal: Increase Muscle Mass and Weight**
There is no point in excessively limiting your rest time. On the contrary, you should give your muscles enough time to fully recover. Trying to lift heavy weights with a muscle that has not fully recovered is counterproductive. However, you should not get carried away and fall asleep during your workout.

A good starting point is to take 45 seconds to 1 minute of rest, depending on your ability to recover. However, resting for more than 2 minutes between sets is excessive.

★ **Goal: Increase Strength**
The heavier you lift, the more rest you will need in order to avoid working a muscle that has not fully recovered. This is why when you are working on increasing your strength, you will need to take longer rest periods.

A good starting point is to take 1 to 2 minutes depending on the weights you lifted. However, 3 minutes is the maximum rest time you should take between sets.

★ **Goal: Increase Power**
Give your muscles at least 30 seconds of rest. One minute is the most rest you should take between sets.

★ **Goal: Improve Isometric Endurance**
Take 30 seconds of rest, maximum, between sets.

★ **Goal: Improve Muscular Endurance**
Rest breaks between sets should be relatively brief (no longer than 30 seconds). The goal here is to work the muscles again before they have a chance to fully recover.

A good strategy is to reduce your rest time gradually over several workouts while trying to maintain (or even increase) the number of repetitions you do. For example, if you did a workout with 30 seconds of rest between sets, then next time you should try to do the same workout while taking only 25 seconds of rest. If, after several sets, you are worn out, then increase the rest time to 30 seconds. During your next workout, try to do even more sets (or even the entire workout) while taking only 25 seconds to rest.

Once you become used to it, the ideal is for you to be able to train in a circuit. This means that you perform several exercises in a row with no real rest time in between. The only break you get is when you are transitioning from one exercise to the next. As you go through your workout and the circuits get harder and harder to do, you can take a 10-second break between each exercise.

## ⑭ What Is the Most Appropriate Weight for Each Movement?

More than the number of repetitions or sets, the resistance (or weight) that you use in each exercise determines the effectiveness of your training. You must use a weight that is suitable for your physical abilities and your goals.

In the beginning, it is often difficult to figure out how much weight to use. Some exercises seem too easy while others seem impossible to do. You might go back and forth a bit, but this is not wasted time. It helps you develop something called muscle memory. To find the right resistance for each exercise, start with a light weight and gradually increase it. There are three broad weight zones:

→ Zone 1 weights are light weights that do not require much effort to lift.
→ Zone 2 weights are weights that allow you both to feel your muscles work and to perform the exercise with good form.
→ Zone 3 weights are heavy weights that require a significant effort to lift them with correct form.

The process for selecting resistance begins with your warm-up. A good warm-up will help you determine the level of resistance. Always start with a light weight.

First, do a warm-up set using a weight from the middle of zone 1. The second preparation set should use a weight from the upper part of zone 1. After that, your goals should determine the weight you lift.

If you do not have a good feel for this, there are some scientifically determined average numbers that you can go by.

Studies by Jidovtseff et al. (2009, *Science and Sports*, 24:91-6) show that an athlete who is using weights that are

→ up to 30% of maximum strength is primarily working on speed,
→ from 30% to 50% of maximum strength is improving power and speed,
→ from 50% to 70% of maximum strength is increasing power and strength, and
→ above 70% of maximum strength is increasing maximum strength.

★ **Goal: Increase Muscle Mass and Weight**
You should use weights from zone 2 for three-quarters of your sets. Gradually increase the weight in each set (pyramid strategy; see page 35). The increase in weight should take you from the lower part of zone 2 to its upper limit.

You can do a final set with a weight from the lower part of zone 3. Handling a weight that is slightly too heavy prepares the nervous system for your next workout. Do not abuse this technique, though, or you could hurt yourself.

★ **Goal: Increase Strength**
After warming up, do your sets with a weight from the lowest part of zone 3. By gradually increasing the weight in each set (pyramid strategy), you will eventually reach the upper part of zone 3.

★ **Goal: Increase Power**
Begin in the lower part of zone 2, and gradually increase the weight in each set until you reach the middle of this same zone.

★ **Goal: Improve Isometric Endurance**
Begin in the middle of zone 3, and gradually increase the duration that you are isometrically contracting the muscles in each set until you reach the top of this same zone.

★ **Goal: Improve Muscular Endurance**

Do your sets with weights from the upper part of zone 1 and the lower part of zone 2. You will not gradually increase the weight because your goal is to fight off the growing fatigue that comes from doing set after set with very little rest time in between.

⚠ **WARNING!**

Remember that you will use different weights for each exercise.

Once you have found the correct weight for an exercise, write it down in a workout notebook along with the number of repetitions you did. When you work out the next time, try to do 1 or 2 more repetitions using the same weight.

## ⑮ When Should You Increase the Weight?

The weight that you can lift for each exercise is constantly changing. In the best case, you get stronger, and this allows you to use heavier and heavier weights. But the natural tendency is to want to jump ahead of this improvement in strength and increase the weight too quickly. This means that your form progressively deteriorates, and you feel less and less work happening in your muscles. Finally, you end up losing your motivation because working out becomes more and more arduous.

Knowing when and how to increase the weight is a critical factor in your progress. There are two criteria that will help you to know whether your muscles are ready for an increase in resistance:

★ 1. **Number of repetitions:** When you surpass the target number of repetitions (12 for muscle mass, for example), it is time to consider increasing your weight.

★ 2. **How easy it is to lift the weight:** If it feels really easy to lift a weight, then you should absolutely increase it.

As a general rule, the increase is only 3 or 5 pounds (~1.5-2.25 kg). It is not useful to add weight faster than that unless you really blew by your target number. In that situation only, you could increase the weight by a larger amount.

♦ **DO NOT ADD WEIGHT TOO FAST**

The more weight you add, the more you risk cheating and using momentum. Sometimes, a small increase in weight is enough to cause a considerable decrease in form. It is better to increase the weight slightly and often, because if you do it abruptly, it could take several workouts to get those muscle sensations back.

♦ **ADJUST YOUR WARM-UP**

As you get stronger, and therefore begin using heavy weights in your first set, your warm-up becomes even more crucial. If you are not very strong, your joints, muscles, and tendons do not need much warming up since the muscle tension required is not very high. As you progress, you will need to increase the number of warm-up sets you do, because the tension you are subjecting your muscles to is gradually approaching their breaking point.

## 16 How Much Rest Time Should You Take Between Exercises?

Between exercises, catch your breath while taking the same amount of time you took between two sets of the same exercise. Increase the time if you feel tired, especially toward the end of a workout. However, you need to move on to the next exercise rather quickly so that you stay focused and your workout does not go on and on.

For circuit training, you should do the exercises with no rest breaks. Ideally, between circuits, you should limit yourself to a small rest break or even take no rest break at all. After a few circuits, when fatigue sets in, start taking 15 to 30 seconds of rest so that you will be able to do 1 or 2 more circuits.

## 17 How Do You Select Exercises Based on Your Anatomomorphology?

In this book, we have carefully selected the most effective exercises for fighters. However, not all of them will necessarily work well for you. Indeed, morphologies differ from person to person. There are tall people, short people, arms and thighs of various sizes, and shoulders of various sizes.

A unique morphology should correspond to an individualized choice of exercises. Not every body type can adapt to every exercise. Certain builds are well suited to some exercises and less so to others. This is the concept of anatomomorphology, the foundation of the Delavier strength training method.

#### ♦ UNEQUAL DIFFICULTY
Since each person's lever length is different, some athletes will have an easier

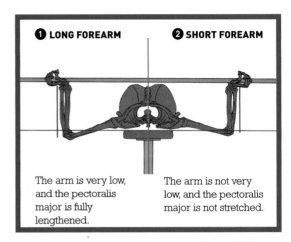

**❶ LONG FOREARM** — The arm is very low, and the pectoralis major is fully lengthened.

**❷ SHORT FOREARM** — The arm is not very low, and the pectoralis major is not stretched.

time than others. For example, a fighter with short arms will have an easier time with narrow-grip bench press since his range of motion is smaller. However, a fighter with long arms will have a harder time because the range of motion is much greater. Even if they use the same weight, the long-armed fighter has to move that weight over a greater distance.

#### ♦ UNEQUAL RISK
As a function of your body type, certain exercises may be more or less dangerous for you. As an example, when doing squats, a fighter with long legs must lean farther forward than a fighter with short thighs. This is not about poor technique when doing an exercise. It is a question of body type. With short thighs, it is relatively easy to keep your back very straight. The longer your thighs are, the more you have to lean forward to maintain your balance. Unfortunately, the farther you lean forward, the greater chance you have of injuring your back.

If you need to take body type into account when selecting an exercise, we note that in the specific description of the exercise.

There are three complementary ways to choose your exercises:

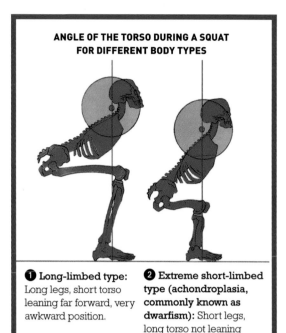

**ANGLE OF THE TORSO DURING A SQUAT FOR DIFFERENT BODY TYPES**

**❶ Long-limbed type:** Long legs, short torso leaning far forward, very awkward position.

**❷ Extreme short-limbed type (achondroplasia, commonly known as dwarfism):** Short legs, long torso not leaning very far forward, not an awkward position.

★ Compound exercises: These are exercises that involve several joints at once. For example, the squat (bending the legs) forces you to move your hips, knees, and ankles.

★ Isolation exercises: These include all exercises that involve only one joint. For example, the biceps curl (bending the forearm over the arm) involves only the elbow joint.

## ⚠ BE CAREFUL ABOUT ISOLATING MUSCLES

Classic strength training exercises tend to focus the work on a single muscle group rather than the whole body. You should avoid these bad habits of focusing on a single muscle group because, during a fight,

→ all of your muscles are under tension, not just a few of them; and

→ the more complex the movement, the more your strength is divided, especially if you are not in the habit of training your body as a whole.

Thus, scientific research has shown that power in the thighs can decrease by up to 40% when the arms are simultaneously contracted compared to when doing an isolation exercise for the thighs.

This strength deficit is only worsened by isolation training. Only total-body strength training (as much as is possible) using compound exercises can fix this problem. **Conclusion:** Programs for fighters should consist mostly of compound exercises. These allow for intense work on a maximum number of muscle groups in a minimum time. Isolation exercises can be added to these basic exercises later on in order to target certain sensitive areas that you want to strengthen (such as neck, forearms, and abdominal muscles).

★ 1. **By elimination:** Some exercises do not work well with your anatomy. You should eliminate those. Other exercises do not work well for the types of strikes you do. These two parameters will restrict the possibilities and make your choices easier. However, simple elimination should not be your only basis for a decision. It is better to find exercises that work well for you.

★ 2. **By selection:** To determine compatibility between your body type and an exercise, often the only way is to try doing the exercise.

★ 3. **By need:** To specifically improve the effectiveness of certain strikes.

♦ **LEARN TO DIFFERENTIATE BETWEEN EXERCISES**

There are two broad categories of exercises. Each has advantages and disadvantages. By choosing exercises from one group rather than another based on your needs, you will make the selection process that much easier.

Compound exercises are more effective than isolation exercises. Indeed, during a fight, muscles work together and not one by one in an isolated manner. If you tried to reproduce the work done through compound exercises using only isolation exercises, you would waste a lot of time. For example, instead of doing a narrow-grip bench press, you would have to do an isolation exercise for the chest muscles plus an exercise for the shoulders plus an exercise for the triceps.

## 18 How Do You Know When to Change Your Program?

Some athletes need to repeat the same workout program. This is easy to understand. After all, once you have found something that works, why change it? Other people need things to stay new and fresh. It is impossible to know beforehand which group you belong to, and most people probably fall somewhere in the middle. But your state of mind generally reflects your muscles' needs fairly accurately. However, there are two objective criteria that indicate when you need to change your workout routine

★ **Plateau or loss of strength:** When your progress abruptly stops, it means that something is no longer working. We are not talking about a single poor workout but a trend over at least one week. A change in your workout is required.
★ **Boredom:** When you lose your enthusiasm for working out, it means that your routine is too monotonous. So you will need to make a change!

♦ CONCLUSION

There is no set rule for when you should change your program. As long as your program is giving you regular results, why change it? There will always come a time when it will be obvious that you should make a change.

## 19 What Time of Day Should You Work Out?

Some people prefer to exercise in the morning, while others prefer the afternoon or evening. In fact, strength varies depending on the time of day. Some people are stronger in the mornings and weaker in the afternoons. For others the opposite is true. These fluctuations are due to the central nervous system and are completely normal. It is rare to find athletes who have consistent strength throughout the day.

Ideally, you should train when your muscles are the strongest. The majority of athletes are strongest around 6 to 7 p.m. This works well since many people have free time to exercise then.

⚠ **WARNING!**

Your workout time may be determined by your daily schedule and not by your body. Even if you are not exercising at your ideal time, a simple rule is that you should always work out at the same time each day. Your muscles will get used to it, and this way they will perform their best at that time.

## 20 How Can You Integrate Strength Training Into Your Fight Training?

Integrating a strength training program into your fighting training is a critical point, especially when you are first beginning with weights. Adding excess work to your fight training will increase your body's need for recovery time and could, at first, cause fatigue.

So it is important not to just start doing strength training whenever you feel like it. There are four ways to incorporate strength training:

★ **Just before fight training:** This is not recommended because muscle fatigue could reduce your ability to practice fighting techniques.

★ **Just after fight training:** Even if you are weaker at this time, this is the easiest way to incorporate strength training into your routine.

★ **In the morning if you do fight training in the afternoon (or vice versa):** You will be less tired when you space out the two workouts, but if you are using very heavy weights, this could lead to overtraining.

★ **On the days when you do not fight:** This is an ideal combination if you have the time and if you do not practice fighting techniques every day.

These four possibilities all have advantages and disadvantages. There is no perfect or universal combination. Within the time available in your schedule, choose the one that is the best for you.

## ROLE OF PERIODIZATION

Periodization is a concept that applies to competitive fighters. It comes from the realization that physical preparation must vary in conjunction with competition dates. Since a sport's season rarely lasts all year, a fighter must perform the best during the competition season. The rest of the time (periods of noncompetition) can be spent on fundamentals or recovery.

Three strategies are available to athletes in the off-season:

→ Reduce the volume of work so you can recover.

→ Use the time to intensify your strength training efforts so that you can boost your performance. This approach allows you to ease up on your weight training once you begin to prepare for competitions.

→ Choose not to periodize your training by trying to make as much progress during the off-season as during the start of competitions. This is the riskiest strategy as far as recovery is concerned.

Choosing one of these strategies is a personal decision. You have to consider your ability to recover and your goals as well as the physical state of your joints, tendons, and muscles.

If you choose to periodize your training, there are three ways to proceed.

### 1 Completely Periodized Training

You choose to stop your training periodically. This phase of total rest can be repeated 1 to 4 times per year. For example, you could take 1 to 2 weeks of rest after 3 consecutive months of strength training.

★ **Advantages:** Muscles and especially joints have time to recover. Mentally, you can relax and begin again with new enthusiasm.

★ **Disadvantages:** It happens frequently that rest weeks turn into months and then years. Stopping and then starting again require discipline, and not everyone is capable of that. It is better for some people to never stop exercising, because then they might never start again. The longer the break, the harder it will be to start again. You must also be very careful about your diet so that you do not gain weight while on a break.

## ❷ Targeted Breaks

Instead of stopping exercise completely, why not shift your focus to one or two muscle groups while simultaneously relaxing your efforts on one or two other muscle groups? For example, you could work your thighs seriously for one month as you lighten up on working your torso. This will give your shoulders and elbows time to recover. The next month, you can focus on your torso as you decrease the amount of work on your thighs.

★ **Advantages:** Rotating muscle groups allows for targeted recovery without causing muscle deconditioning, which is what would happen if you stopped training completely. No effort is required to begin exercising again, and there is little risk of gaining any weight. You will not waste any time with superfluous rest periods.

★ **Disadvantages:** You are constantly on the edge without any chance to take a mental break. This strategy is currently the default strategy when dealing with injuries. If your knee is hurting, you stop working your thighs, and you really go to work on your torso instead.

## ❸ No Breaks

This is the simplest and most popular strategy. Effort is continually maintained. As long as you are not overtraining, why stop? You will need to sharpen your skills only just before competitions begin.

★ **Advantages:** If you pace yourself, you will continue to make progress without wasting any time or regressing during rest periods.

★ **Disadvantages:** The joints do not have time to recover, and it is generally too late once you start to have problems with them.

◆ **CONCLUSION**

You will have to choose a strategy based on your ability to recover. The inherent weakness in taking breaks is that you have to guess how your body will react in the future. You make these predictions based on things that happened in the past, and chances are high that you could make a mistake.

Our philosophy toward taking breaks is simple: When you are feeling strong, take advantage and go all out during your workouts. There will certainly be other workouts where you will not physically be able to do this.

# TECHNIQUES FOR INCREASING STRENGTH AND POWER

You can use many techniques to gain strength, but not all of them are appropriate for fighting. Some may even be counterproductive for a fighter. Here we have selected only the most effective techniques for fighting sports.

## EIGHT PRINCIPLES TO PREPARE THE MUSCLES FOR FIGHTING

It is understood that when you do strength training, the strength you gain in the gym will translate into improved performance in the ring. For a beginner, this transfer generally happens well. But the more experienced you are as a fighter, the more problematic this transfer becomes.

To ensure an optimal transfer, your strength training needs to develop those physical qualities that are required in a fight. This is why it is imperative that you stick to these eight principles as faithfully as possible.

### 1 Fight Conditions

Many of the most popular strength training exercises do not correspond well to the strikes used in a fight. One such exercise is the wide-grip bench press. Though this exercise will really help a beginner who is not very strong, it is not well suited for an experienced fighter. This is because it is rare to throw a punch while your shoulder blades are stabilized on a bench or on the floor. To optimize your fighting ability while standing, you should do strength training exercises while standing up and without supporting your shoulder blades.

### 2 Direction of Movement

If you are a beginner and want to do bench presses, you need to avoid the common mistake of using a wide grip as in classic strength training. A wide grip does not correlate with the kinds of strikes used during fights, since you rarely hit on the outside of the body. You must adjust your grip to the width of your strikes. In other words, you should use a narrow grip.

### 3 Direction of Strength

When you throw a punch, you have to overcome horizontal resistance. It would not be useful to box with dumbbells, because they provide vertical resistance. Using an elastic band that is parallel to the floor or a cable machine is much more appropriate.

### 4 The Sides of the Body Used in a Fight

Going back to the example of the bench press, it is an exercise that is done with both arms at the same time. But since fighters do not punch with both fists at the same time, it is better to do presses with only one arm at a time. However, once you knock an opponent down, you do use both arms together, and this closely matches the action in a deadlift. Choking an opponent on the ground with your thighs is always a bilateral movement. Therefore, you should choose strength training exercises on a case-by-case basis depending on which sides of the body are used in the exercise.

## 5 Range of Motion in Movements

Strength training exercises should mirror the range of motion used in your fighting moves.

It is not helpful to do exercises with a greater range of motion. Rather, you can do exercises with a slightly smaller range of motion because they will help you get stronger without necessarily constituting the majority of your workout.

## 6 Types of Muscle Contraction Necessary in a Fight

Classic strength training exercises mainly have a back-and-forth rhythm of contraction. This harmonious succession correlates perfectly with running sports, for example. But, during a fight, the series of moves happen with much less certainty, often with a few seconds of rest between blows. So you need to practice this style of random moves.

## 7 Speed of Execution

How quickly you move your weights while you are strength training should match what you do in a fight: explosive so you can throw a punch; using a little more strength when you want to knock an opponent down or flip him over; isometric (with almost no movement) for many holds done on the ground, such as locks, chokes, and defensive moves. So you should use many different speeds during your workouts.

## 8 Types of Strength Required in a Fight

Strength is a generic term that encompasses many realities. It is a good idea to analyze the primary movements in a fight so you can define which muscle qualities you need to develop first.

---

## FIVE TYPES OF STRENGTH MOST OFTEN USED IN FIGHTING

You need to develop five types of strength as a fighter:

## 1 Maximum Strength

You must reach a critical level of strength that will allow you to contain an opponent, especially if you have not mastered many techniques. It is better for you to give your opponent the impression that he is about to face a steamroller than to feel as if your opponent is the steamroller. The weights you lift in strength training should be heavier than what you encounter in a fight.

## 2 Initial Strength

To throw a punch or prepare for an attack, your muscles have to react immediately. Besides reflexes, the speed of your strikes depends on how fast your strength propagates through your muscles. This is a muscle quality that you have to cultivate (in the box titled "Understanding Rate of Force Development" on page 33).

The power of your blows depends on the rate of force development (RFD), or how quickly strength propagates through the muscle. Good RFD allows for rapid diffusion of strength through the muscles.

Imagine that you have to throw a small ball. The difficulty is not the weight of the ball since it is very light, but your ability to quickly mobilize your maximum strength to throw the ball. This ability is what makes someone good at throwing, because once the thrower initiates the movement, there is very little time before his arm is straight and the ball is thrown. Someone who cannot throw a ball very far is not weak; his propagation speed is just too slow. This means that his arm cannot transfer much power to the ball.

This type of person generally performs better when using a heavier ball. Because the ball weighs more, the movement is slower. This allows more time for the thrower's strength to propagate through the muscle. It is the same for a punch. In boxing, a good punch is thrown in 50 to 250 milliseconds.

But a muscle requires 600 to 800 milliseconds to attain its maximum strength. A sedentary person can, on average, recruit 15% of his strength in 50 milliseconds, but a good athlete can recruit 26% of his strength in that time (Tillin et al., 2010, *Medicine and Science in Sport and Exercise,* 42:781-90). This is because a champion athlete has an RFD that is twice as high as that of the average person.

Once your arm starts to move, there is very little time to mobilize your strength and throw the punch. Only a fraction of your total strength can be expressed in less than 250 milliseconds. Athletes who strike the hardest have the highest RFD. This quality depends in large part on the nervous systems (genetics), but it can be improved through training, especially through strength training.

If you can transfer only 15% of your strength in a punch, then you can make that punch more effective by increasing your maximum strength. If you increase your maximum strength from 100 pounds to 200 pounds, then your punch will be twice as powerful even with a poor RFD. The ideal, of course, is to increase your maximum strength and RFD simultaneously.

For beginners, 14 weeks of strength training using heavy weights that allow for 3 to 10 repetitions accelerates RFD by

→ 23% for a contraction lasting less than 50 milliseconds, and

→ 17% for the following 100 to 200 milliseconds.

Maximum strength increases by 16% (Aagaard et al., 2002, *Journal of Applied Physiology,* 93(6):2309-18).

There are techniques for increasing intensity that are more precise than just using heavy weights, and these will help develop your RFD. (See Improving Isometric Strength on page 39.)

## ③ Isometric Strength

To block or choke an opponent or put him in a submission, your muscles must be strong and have endurance during a static contraction.

## ④ Explosive Plyometric Strength

This is seen in your ability to wind up (footwork or pulling your arm or leg back before you strike or throw a kick). Indeed, the farther back you pull your arm or leg before a strike, the more obvious your intended strike will be to your opponent.

## ⑤ Dynamic Muscular Endurance

You cannot afford to be strong for just one minute. A fighter has to conserve as much strength as possible through all the rounds, and this is made possible by developing muscular endurance (see the sections starting on page 41).

### ♦ CONCLUSION

You need to evaluate how much you use each of these kinds of strength in your fighting techniques. Your strength training program should include work for each of these types of strength in order of their respective importance. We will now discuss the most effective ways to increase intensity so you can develop these types of strength.

## SECRETS OF AN EFFECTIVE STRIKE

To be effective, a broad strike happens in three phases:

★ 1. **A rapid but short muscle contraction** initiates the most violent movement possible.
★ 2. **Muscle relaxation** causes the arm or thigh to gain speed and range of motion without hindrance from antagonistic muscles (biceps and upper back muscles that slow down a punch or hamstrings and gluteals that slow down a kick).
★ 3. **Contracting the muscle again** just before impact produces the critical force that will do the most damage possible.

### Practical Consequences of Strength Training

In strength training, it is difficult to reproduce this three-part sequence using only one technique to increase intensity. So that you do not hinder the transfer of your increased strength and power, it is a good idea to combine several techniques to increase intensity. Do not restrict yourself to working only with heavy weights. Even though using increasing amounts of resistance is an effective way to increase the strength of your blows, it is not a perfect strategy. Since there is no intermediate relaxation phase, ultimately, heavy weights will interfere with the motor learning for your strikes.

This imperfection explains why scientific research shows that working exclusively with heavy weights ends up decreasing the speed of a fighter's strikes after 12 to 18 weeks (Siff, 1999, *Supertraining*). This is why you should not depend solely on heavy training to achieve progress.

### How Can You Improve the Qualities Required for an Effective Strike?

Only by judiciously combining these various techniques to increase intensity will you improve the three phases that make a strike effective:

★ 1. **Heavy weights** increase strength and therefore the effectiveness of the strike initially and on impact.
★ 2. **Stop-and-go work using elastic bands** increases the speed with which your strength propagates through the muscle.
★ 3. **Explosive training with average weights** increases the speed of muscle relaxation.

Ideally, you should end the explosive contraction phase by actually hitting something so you can maintain the sequence and end by contracting the muscle again. In fact, when you practice explosive technique with weights or just by doing shadow boxing, your own antagonistic muscles stop your fist or your foot. These two techniques actually work against the contraction–relaxation cycle just described. They are also counterproductive in regard to the final phase where the muscle contracts again just before impact. In fact, contracting the antagonistic muscles to stop your punch actually teaches you not to hit as hard as possible upon impact.

To reduce the degree to which strength training causes neuromuscular disturbance in your strikes, it is a good idea to end your workouts by spending a few minutes hitting a punching bag.

## Working With a Half Pyramid

A set of strength training exercises is designed around a half pyramid. You should start with modest resistance and a high number of repetitions (25, for example, that are easy to do) to warm up the muscles, joints, and cardiorespiratory system thoroughly. For the second set, you should increase the weight so you can easily do 15 repetitions. These two warm-up sets help to precondition your muscles.

Then the serious work begins: Add resistance until you reach the upper range of the target number of repetitions that you set as a function of your goals. As you keep doing sets, gradually increase the resistance to make the exercise harder. The number of repetitions will decrease as you continue. When the weight is so heavy that you can no longer reach the lower range of your target number of repetitions, it is time to move on to another exercise.

In bodybuilding, it is common to decrease the weight in the last set so that you can do 15 to 20 more repetitions to get the muscles pumped up as much as possible. But getting pumped up would be a catastrophe for a fighter, so it is wise to train using the half pyramid model (you only increase the weight) rather the pyramid model (where you increase the weight and then decrease it).

## BREATHING DURING STRENGTH TRAINING

Breathing affects your performance:
→ Holding your breath lets your muscles express their full power.
→ Exhaling slightly decreases your strength.
→ Inhaling seriously weakens your muscles.

These physiological responses are perfectly illustrated in the strategies that champion arm wrestlers use. They wait for their opponent to inhale, and then they hold their breath in order to unleash their full strength and win the match. In other words, they mobilize their full power by holding their breath at the exact moment that their opponent is at his weakest (because he inhaled).

Holding the breath is a natural reflex. Strength, reaction time, precision of movement, and concentration are all briefly improved when you hold your breath. Another advantage of breath holding is that it rigidifies the spine. This protects the lumbar region when the back is under a great deal of pressure.

## Breathing During Heavy Work

The more you lift heavy weights, the more you will need to use breath holding to improve your performance. Ideally, you should hold your breath as briefly as possible. You should hold your breath briefly when the exercise is the hardest. For example, when you work your biceps by bringing your hands toward your shoulders, the hardest part of the exercise is when the forearms are parallel to the floor. Before and after this angle, the exercise is easier. It would be counterproductive to hold your breath the entire time you are lifting the weight; you need to do it only during the fraction of a second when your arms are parallel. But you should not ever inhale at that moment. Inhale deeply between repetitions or during the easiest part of the exercise (lowering the weight).

## Clenching Your Teeth Gives You Power

Muscles are designed to work together, not separately. Therefore, it is not surprising that people are naturally inclined to tense up when strength training exercises get hard. Scientific research has shown that strength increases by about 5% when you clench your teeth. It is the same when you clench your fists.

One reason for this is that nervous system reflexes are increased (Jendrassik maneuver). This is particularly apparent in the thighs, with an increase of 19% in the RFD; in the arms, there is a 15% increase (Ebben et al., 2008. *Journal of Strength and Conditioning Research* 22(6):1850-54).

## ADAPTING STRENGTH TRAINING TO THE DEMANDS OF A FIGHT

For optimal transfer, strength training must adapt to a fighter's needs, not the other way around. Compared to strength training exercises, the blows used in a fight are very different:

→ The rhythm of strikes is jerky, but strength training is very rhythmic.
→ Rest periods between two blows are random, but in strength training, repetitions are done one after the other without much rest.
→ A fighter does everything possible to rid the body of lactic acid and to avoid pumping up the muscles, but a bodybuilder strives for both burn and pump.

To overcome this triple difference, two techniques for increasing intensity are appropriate:

### ❶ Stop and Go to Accelerate Initial Strength

This technique involves pausing for 1 to 2 seconds between each repetition. For example, when doing push-ups, you stay elongated on the floor for 1 second while you relax the muscles and then activate them, causing the contraction. The goal of this pause is to eliminate the accumulation of elastic energy that took place during the lowering phase of the push-up.

You must pause at the bottom of the exercise rather than the top so that the repetition begins with a positive phase (pushing the weight) rather than a negative phase (lowering) because this is how you strike blows against your opponent.

The stop-and-go technique benefits a fighter in these ways:

★ 1. **It is very useful for improving initial strength.** The muscles have to contract powerfully without the benefit of elastic energy stored up during the negative phase.

★ 2. **It is important to work on the initial strength of a muscle in a near-resting state** rather than a muscle that is already contracted, since this is very rare in a fight.

★ 3. **The combined work** of initial strength and acceleration strength will help you become quicker.

★ 4. **The rhythmic tempo of repetitions** in classic strength training promotes blood flow, which is not good. The staccato rhythm of the stop-and-go pauses will minimize pump and the accumulation of lactic acid.

★ 5. **A random tempo** mimics the conditions in a fight better than classic strength training does.

## ② Doing Sets With a Between-Reps Break

The natural tendency is to want to do repetitions as quickly as possible one after the other. This bodybuilding tactic is not ideal for a fighter. When repetitions come without pause, fatigue quickly sets in because the blood flow is hindered. Metabolic wastes, such as lactic acid, build up and cause strength to decrease.

Furthermore, the muscle starts to get pumped up. If you train your muscles to get pumped up the way bodybuilders do, you will paralyze yourself more easily during fights.

So you need to do whatever you can so that your muscles do not get in the habit of getting pumped up. A pause between each repetition minimizes the pump caused by the restriction of blood flow. Blood circulates more freely, which helps transport oxygen and allows you to stay stronger for longer periods.

### ⚠ BE CAREFUL OF MUSCLE FAILURE

The philosophy of between-reps breaks consists of doing everything you can to avoid fatigue instead of seeking it out as you would in bodybuilding. To be able to work out a lot without wearing yourself out, you would be well advised to avoid failure (temporary fatigue of the neuromuscular system). As Charlie Francis, former trainer of sprinter Ben Johnson, notes, a 100% effort requires 10 days of recovery time. But if you push to only 95% of your ability, just 4 hours of recovery time is needed between two workouts.

This explains why scientific research shows that it is not a good idea for beginners to push sets until failure. Striving for failure is more appropriate for those working on muscle mass than for those wanting to increase strength or power.

Between-reps recovery breaks let you work with as heavy a weight as you can without exhausting your nervous system for a long time afterward. Thus, you can do your various workouts more closely together while still minimizing the risk of physically exhausting yourself.

Taking 15 seconds of rest between each repetition allows your muscles to recover up to 80% of their initial strength (Haff et al., 2003, *Journal of Strength and Conditioning Research* 17(1):95-103). With the same weight and a similar rest break, spacing out the repetitions instead of doing them one right after the other immediately increases strength by 30% (Denton and Cronin, 2006, *Journal of Strength and Conditioning Research* 20(3):528-34).

By resting for 15 to 20 seconds between 2 repetitions (midset break), you can lift heavier weights and get stronger faster.

## Plyometric Workouts

Explosive training with light weights (about 30% of the maximum weight you can lift) has two advantages for a fighter:

→ It improves power, since these weights optimize the speed of muscle contraction.
→ It increases the capacity for muscle relaxation during a movement.

In fact, the difference between experienced fighters and beginners is the speed of muscle relaxation, which is 8 times faster in champion fighters. For an inexperienced fighter, the speed of muscle relaxation is too slow for the leg or the fist to gain enough speed when striking a blow. Keeping the antagonistic muscles contracted automatically slows down the movement.

This muscle conflict slows down the impact, reducing the effectiveness of the attack and facilitating the opponent's escape. Plyometric training helps you accelerate the speed of muscle relaxation after a powerful contraction. However, heavy work is still very appropriate for improving a short strike during which there is no relaxation phase.

## Advantages of Training With Elastic Bands

The resistance provided by an elastic band is very different than that provided by a dumbbell. The more you pull on an elastic band, the more the resistance increases. However, when you lift a 20-pound dumbbell, it will always weigh 20 pounds whether you are at the beginning, middle, or end of the movement.

Elastic bands, by providing increasing resistance,
→ develop acceleration strength,
→ inhibit the intervention of antagonistic muscles that slow down strikes, and
→ improve strength upon impact.

Furthermore, the feeling of resistance provided by an elastic band varies depending on the position of the band. The band could therefore be horizontal, vertical, or at 45 degrees, not just vertical as with a dumbbell.

Fighters who spend eight weeks working on punches using elastic bands as resistance accelerate the speed of the punch by 17% (Dinn and Behm, 2007, *International Journal of Sports Physiology and Performance.* 2:386-99).

However, elastic bands do inhibit the intermediate relaxation sequence, which means that you should not train exclusively with bands. Otherwise you could interfere with the motor learning for your strikes.

♦ **CONCLUSION**

You should not compare the resistance provided by bands to that provided by weights. Both have advantages; one is not better than the other. Ideally, you should alternate between them or use both so that you get the most benefit from each kind of resistance. In the second part of this book, we show you a great number of exercises that you can do with elastic bands alone or with elastic bands plus weights.

## Improving Isometric Strength

For combat sports that take place partly or completely on the ground or against a cage, static muscular endurance (also called isometric strength) is essential. Isometric means a muscle contraction that combines strength and endurance. If your sport includes this, then you absolutely have to focus on it in your training.

Static, or isometric, strength has two forms:

★ 1. **Offensive isometrics:** You grab your opponent in order to hold him, choke him, or make him submit. To improve your abilities, you should do a lot of static contractions for the chest and biceps.

★ 2. **Defensive isometrics:** You resist the holds your opponent tries to use by pressing against the floor or the cage. If your opponent is stronger than you are, you will move from a static to a negative contraction, which signals that you are about to lose the fight. So that this does not happen to you, you need to work your back, shoulders, and triceps through static exercises.

But the key muscles, whether for defense or offense, are the adductors and the muscles in the front of the lower legs (tibialis anterior). These are the only two muscle groups that you should train exclusively with static exercises.

Isometrics during a fight happen in two phases:

★ 1. **Explosive isometrics:** On contact, it is best to be able to mobilize 100% of your strength as fast as possible. Working on RFD is very important so that your opponent has the shortest time to get out of your grip or to secure his own grip. You should work on explosive isometrics as opposed to slow isometrics in which resistance increases gradually (for example, a rugby match where the tension between opponents mounts in a crescendo before the ball is thrown in). To do this, use weights that are heavier than your maximum and try to push them up with brutality and fury.

★ 2. **Isometric endurance** then takes over. The first fighter who gets tired is in the weaker position. So you should train yourself to maintain an isometric contraction as long as possible (at least 30 seconds).

Begin with explosive contractions that you hold for 5 to 10 seconds. In future workouts, you can gradually increase the amount of time you hold the contractions.

→ **If you are weak in explosive isometrics,** you should take 15 to 30 seconds to rest between repetitions so that you can really work on the strength of the muscle while it is as fresh as possible.

→ **If you are weak in isometric endurance,** take as short a rest break as possible (5 to 10 seconds) between repetitions so that you can work that tired muscle again.

In both cases, a single set per exercise that includes the maximum number of repetitions will be sufficient. The set should end when you feel your strength ebbing.

Your goal for the next workout is to do at least 1 more repetition before you are exhausted. Ideally, you should do isometric sets toward the end of your workout once you are already tired. The goal here is to reproduce as faithfully as you can the physiological conditions you experience in a fight.

The angle you use when doing isometric work should be as close as possible to the angle used in your fighting style. For example, for free fighting, the adductors are often worked with the thighs open to 45 degrees each, not with the thighs squeezed together.

You need to be especially attentive to your breathing during isometrics. Holding your breath briefly increases your strength quickly so that you can grab your opponent. But if you hold your breath longer, you will not get enough oxygen. So you have to learn to breathe without negatively affecting your muscle strength. You should practice this technique every time you do strength training exercises.

## Should You Exercise in an Unstable Environment?

Training in an unstable environment is popular at the moment. For example, instead of doing a bench press on a bench (stable surface), it is recommended that you do it while lying on an exercise ball (or Swiss ball), which is an unstable surface. This method, which comes from physical therapy, allows you to do the following:

→ Reduce the amount of weight you lift in order to minimize stress on your joints.
→ Better balance the strength in the muscles on your right side with those on your left side.

What about fighters? In a fight, the floor is always stable, and your opponent is what causes instability. Scientific studies show that to improve balance, the conditions you train in should closely mirror those you encounter in your particular sport (Keogh et al., 2010, *Journal of Strength and Conditioning Research,* 24(2):422-29). Fighting has nothing in common with practicing strength training on an unstable surface.

This explains why, with the exception of sliding sports, training on an unstable surface slows gains in strength instead of augmenting them. Compared to an exercise done on a stable surface, strength decreases by 22% on an unstable surface (Kohler et al., 2010, *Journal of Strength and Conditioning Research,* 24(2):313-21). Because of this loss, the supporting muscles, which are supposed to work more on an unstable surface, are in fact recruited 34% less. Therefore, instability is not a good idea if you want to gain as much strength as you can in as short a time as possible.

Unless one day fighters were to compete on a giant exercise ball, they will gain very little by training in an unstable environment. Furthermore, it is pointless and dangerous to handle heavy weights while perched on a moveable surface. Once you hurt yourself by falling, you will see how much progress you have made!

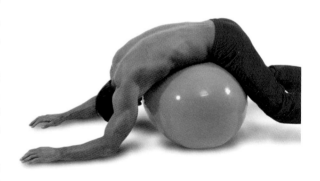

Though it is useful for relaxing the back muscles by promoting vertebral decompression, the exercise ball is not recommended for fighters doing strength training.

# TECHNIQUES FOR IMPROVING CONDITIONING AND ENDURANCE

It does no good for you as a fighter to be strong and powerful and to thoroughly master fighting techniques if you lack endurance. This quality is indispensable and has to be developed through conditioning techniques.

## POWER AND CONDITIONING: TWO VERY DIFFERENT MUSCLE QUALITIES

Muscles were designed to specialize in one kind of work, either power or endurance, but not both. Performing strength training regularly increases the number of fast-twitch muscle fibers (type 2). And the distribution of muscle fibers is not fixed; it constantly changes depending on the kind of work the muscles are required to do. Mathematically, a gain in strength fibers means that the muscles are losing endurance, or slow-twitch (type 1) fibers.

Slow- and fast-twitch fibers are not something you can see with the naked eye. But, on average, the RFD of type 2 fibers is twice as fast as that of type 1 fibers. For a punch that lasts only 50 to 250 milliseconds, the difference in effectiveness will be noticeable. This power in type 2 fibers occurs to the detriment of their ability to resist fatigue, because they tire out very quickly. On the contrary, even though type 1 fibers are slower, they can endure far longer. Doing cardio training will help increase resistance, but it could also decrease your power.

This opposition helps explain why it is difficult to have both power and endurance. Still, as a fighter you need both qualities in order to win. To achieve this, you should do circuit training. Circuit training involves doing a variety of strength training exercises in a row with no rest breaks between sets.

## FIVE RULES FOR MINIMIZING OPPOSITION OF POWER AND ENDURANCE

### 1 You Are Not Rocky

Certainly, never-ending jogging sessions may seem like a good idea at first, but they are not. They will limit your power for no good reason.

### 2 Avoid Cardio Training That Lasts Longer Than the Time You Spend in a Fight

Unlike many sports where the length of time you spend in a competition is unknown (tennis, for example), the maximum length of a fight is known in advance. You need to base the length of your cardio training on this number.

### ❸ Mimic the Rest Break Intervals in a Fight

There is no point in a circuit that lasts longer than a single round. For example, for MMA, try to do 3 circuits of exercises, spending 5 minutes for each circuit, with a 1-minute rest break in between circuits. The goal is to develop the same energy channels as those required during a fight.

### ❹ Work the Entire Body

The problem with classic cardio exercises is that they are repetitive and they do not stimulate all the muscles in the body. Often, they focus only on the lower body (running, biking, treadmill, step) instead of the entire body. This is why circuit training is essential. With dumbbells, you are using greater resistance than just your body weight, which makes your conditioning workout even more effective and works your entire body.

### ❺ First, Develop Your Strength

After focusing on gaining strength for several weeks, you should gradually start doing more conditioning work. Beyond a certain level, the transfer of strength, in terms of actual progress in the ring, will diminish. Once you have doubled the amount of weight you lift (for the strongest fighters before they began strength training) or tripled it (for fighters who were not as strong), you will make more progress by improving your conditioning than by focusing on pure strength.

## ADJUSTING CIRCUITS FOR OPTIMAL CONDITIONING

Thinking about neuromuscular ability, you should be able to go from a maximum muscle contraction in the arms to one in the thighs, or even do both at the same time, and all in a completely random order and without the muscles' having any time to adapt. This is the benefit of circuit training, since it prepares you for these abrupt and random variations.

In classic strength training, the muscles are artificially segmented. You do several sets of the same exercise before moving on to a new exercise. A fight does not happen this way.

Strength training in circuits lets you constantly change the exercise and, therefore, the muscle groups. These continual changes in exercises are closer to what is required in the ring than a classic strength training workout.

In many sports, the benefit of a circuit is that it is logical. In fighting, the benefit of a circuit is that there is no set order given the large variety of movements needed in a fight.

♦ **CONCLUSION**
Circuits are ideal for developing functional muscular endurance. They also give you a shorter workout since there is little rest time.

## Circuits and Mental Preparation

During strength training, it is not just your muscles that are working hard; your brain is also controlling the muscle contractions. Scientific research has shown that the regions of the brain that are working when you do classic sets are different than when you are doing circuits.

When you do classic sets, repeating the same movement allows your brain a certain amount of rest. When you do circuits, the constant change in motor recruitment requires the brain to keep alert. This is harder for your brain, but it trains your brain to increase its performance during complex tasks that require random muscle recruitment, such as in a fight.

## Developing a Circuit

A beginner typically cannot do a circuit for several minutes using heavy weights. Start by taking 15 to 30 seconds of rest between exercises in a circuit. As you continue working out, reduce the rest time until you no longer need any rest at all. Examples of circuits are provided in part 3 of this book (beginning on page 126).

## Breathing During Endurance Work

When you are doing circuit training, you need to breathe as much as possible to keep your body oxygenated. In this case, it is better to avoid holding your breath despite the natural temptation to do so. Exhale during the hardest part of the exercise (lifting the weight) and inhale during the easiest part (lowering the weight).

## HOW TO DEAL WITH LACTIC ACID

The acidification of muscles is a direct indication of fatigue. During a fight, the production of lactic acid can be multiplied by 10. There is a simple way to render this acid inactive and reduce any loss of performance. Just use a supplement that is a base, such as baking soda, which neutralizes the acid.

In one study, high-level boxers took 300 milligrams of baking soda per kilogram (approximately 2 pounds) of body weight 90 minutes before a fight (4 rounds lasting 3 minutes each, with 1 minute of rest in between) (Siegler and Hirscher, 2010, *Journal of Strength and Conditioning Research,* 24(1):103-8). Taking the baking soda just before the fight made the boxers' blood less acidic (pH 7.43) than those who took a placebo (pH 7.37), which meant they started the fight with a definite advantage.

At the end of the fight, the blood was still less acidic due to the baking soda (pH 7.22 versus 7.17 with placebo). Since the lactic acid did not paralyze the muscles as much, performance was improved. Concretely, the baking soda allowed a 5% increase in the number of blows struck during the entire fight. The difference becomes noticeable in the third round and is even more evident in the fourth round.

This example shows that nutrition and supplementation play an important role in a fighter's development.

# TECHNIQUES FOR INCREASING FLEXIBILITY

## FLEXIBILITY AND STIFFNESS: TWO OPPOSITE MUSCLE QUALITIES

In theory, muscle stiffness is seen as a defect, while flexibility is seen as an asset. Unfortunately, things are much more complex than that.

For a fighter, flexibility provides many advantages:

→ Flexible muscles are a prerequisite for numerous strikes, especially those done with the legs.

→ Being flexible, or even hyperflexible, is the best line of defense against submission techniques.

→ Having a good range of motion in your joints can help you escape from many holds more easily.

→ Flexibility helps you maintain your balance better; it is easy to knock a stiff fighter off balance.

→ A flexible muscle is less likely than a stiff muscle to be injured.

However, there is a flip side to this:

→ Too much flexibility decreases muscle power. The least flexible among high-level athletes have a 37% higher RFD than those who are more flexible.

→ Hyperflexibility can compromise endurance.

→ To protect your torso from blows, it is better to be a little bit stiff.

### Striking a Balance Between Flexibility and Stiffness

All athletic disciplines must deal with this conflict between flexibility and stiffness. In certain activities, it is easy to resolve this dilemma: For dancers, flexibility is crucial. In strength sports, stiffness is more important. The problem for you as a fighter is that you must combine the flexibility of a dancer and the stiffness of a very strong man.

However, keep in mind that flexibility is not an end in and of itself. It is just one more way to fight better. Of course, being really flexible is impressive, but beyond a certain point, too much flexibility will render your strikes less effective.

It is a good idea to find a compromise between stiffness and flexibility in a muscle. This balance was defined by the Soviet bodybuilding masters: A muscle needs to stay flexible enough to have a slightly larger range of motion than is required in your athletic discipline (to prevent injuries and so that stiffness does not interfere with your movements), but not much more (so your performance is not diminished and you do not become like a rag doll whose joints move too easily).

### ♦ CONCLUSION

We can deduce from all of this that stretching a muscle can either increase or decrease its performance. You need to pay attention and learn to stretch correctly.

## Flexible Muscles Are Not Flexible Joints

Doing the splits, both front and side, is seen as a sign of flexibility. But just because you can do the splits does not mean that you are flexible. And if you cannot do the splits, it does not mean that you are not flexible.

In fact, not all morphologies were made to do the splits.

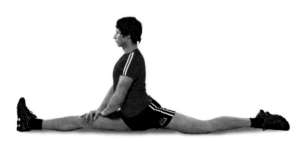

Doing the splits is more a question of morphology than flexibility.

### ♦ CONCLUSION

Your bone structure plays an important role in your range of motion. Making your muscles and tendons more flexible is one thing. Hurting your bones by forcing them to do movements for which they were not made (just because some people can do those movements) is another thing entirely. This kind of stubbornness will only cause you unnecessary pain. From this morphological example, we can glean two commonsense rules that will help you avoid pain and injury:

★ 1. **Focus on strikes and blows that are suitable** for your bone and ligament structure.

★ 2. **Adapt your strength training workouts** to your morphology.

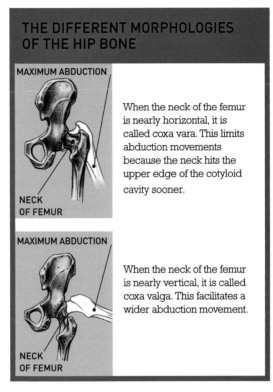

**THE DIFFERENT MORPHOLOGIES OF THE HIP BONE**

MAXIMUM ABDUCTION

When the neck of the femur is nearly horizontal, it is called coxa vara. This limits abduction movements because the neck hits the upper edge of the cotyloid cavity sooner.

NECK OF FEMUR

MAXIMUM ABDUCTION

When the neck of the femur is nearly vertical, it is called coxa valga. This facilitates a wider abduction movement.

NECK OF FEMUR

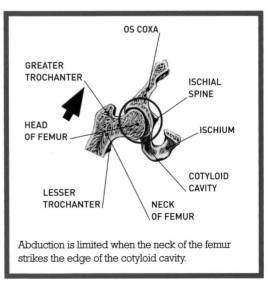

OS COXA

GREATER TROCHANTER

ISCHIAL SPINE

HEAD OF FEMUR

ISCHIUM

LESSER TROCHANTER

NECK OF FEMUR

COTYLOID CAVITY

Abduction is limited when the neck of the femur strikes the edge of the cotyloid cavity.

## Strength Training and Muscle Stiffness

Strength training with heavy weights tends to reduce the flexibility of a muscle. This is normal because muscles require a certain amount of stiffness in order to be strong and powerful.

But this can ultimately reduce your range of motion, which will decrease your performance. It can also cause injuries. Stretching regularly can minimize this problem.

## Enhanced Flexibility With Unilateral Stretching

You are more flexible when you stretch one limb at a time (unilateral stretching) than when you stretch both your right and left sides simultaneously (bilateral stretching). This physiological characteristic highlights the role of the nervous system in your ability to stretch. Instinctively, you might think that only muscle–tendon flexibility determines the range of motion. However, bilateral stretching demonstrates that protection by the nervous system happens much earlier than with unilateral stretching, and this restricts the range of motion. If you are trying to increase your range of motion quickly, you would benefit more by doing unilateral stretching first instead of bilateral stretching. These are also the kinds of stretches most often observed in fighting.

### ♦ CONCLUSION

The key to flexibility is in the central nervous system. Efficient regulation of tension in the muscles and tendons by the nervous system allows you to have both stiffness (when you have to strike hard) and flexibility. You can achieve this malleability and adaptability of the nervous system only through a combination of strength training with heavy weights and regular stretching exercises.

## WHEN TO STRETCH

There are four occasions for developing flexibility:

###  During the Warm-Up

If you stretch out a rubber band for a few seconds, it will get warm. This same phenomenon of tension being transformed into heat happens in your muscles when you stretch them. This is why stretching warms up muscles and tendons. If you pull too hard on the rubber band, it will get too stretched out and lose its tension. Even worse, it could tear. The same thing can happen with muscles, which are just like giant rubber bands.

Always do warm-up stretching gently. In fact, scientific research indicates that stretching warm-ups can diminish performance due to decreased muscle elasticity. Losing even a small amount of reactivity makes a muscle less explosive and less powerful, and it will therefore have less endurance. This decrease in performance is temporary, but it lasts long enough to interfere with a strength training workout or a fight. So do not push your stretches too far during a warm-up. Warm-up stretching is only supposed to warm up the muscle; it is not supposed to increase flexibility.

## 2 While Exercising

Strength training and practicing fighting techniques are fragmented activities. This means you can stretch during breaks. At that moment, stretching can have two effects:

1. In the best case, stretching allows you to regain muscle tone quickly by enhancing recovery, which translates to an improvement in performance.
2. In the worst case, stretching can accentuate fatigue.

Both of these extreme responses can be explained and are not as surprising as they first appear. They depend in large part on the degree of muscle fatigue as well as the type of stretching you are doing. It might even happen that stretching proves beneficial during the first part of a workout and then counterproductive at the end of the workout. The opposite can also happen.

The advantage of stretching is that you immediately feel its benefits or any potential negative effects.

Do not feel that you have to stretch during every workout. Even if some people love to do it, it does not benefit every person in every situation.

## 3 Immediately After Working Out

This is a good time to stretch, because there is no way you will suffer from any potential temporary decrease in performance. In addition, your muscles are already nice and warm. But here are the disadvantages of this strategy:

→ It increases your total workout time.
→ Stretching muscles while they are tired is not ideal for quickly increasing flexibility.

However, if you just want to maintain your level of flexibility, the postworkout period is an ideal time to stretch.

## 4 Between Workouts, on Rest Days

If you need to increase your flexibility quickly, you should do this until you reach your desired level of flexibility. The advantage of stretching is that you can do it at home without the need for much equipment. The disadvantage is that these stretching workouts add to your total number of workouts as well as your volume of work, which could slow down your recovery.

The other problem inherent in this strategy is that you are working the muscle when it is cold, which could be risky. So remember these tactics:

→ Warm up well before you stretch.
→ Gradually increase the length of your stretches.

The two main types of stretching are static and dynamic.

## ❶ Static Stretching

Static stretching means holding the stretch for 10 seconds to 1 minute. The degree of stretch can be from light to strong depending on your goals.

★ **Advantages:** Practiced in a controlled and progressive manner, static stretching is the least likely to cause an injury.

★ **Disadvantages:** This type of stretching is most likely to cause a decrease in performance when done just before a workout.

## ❷ Dynamic Stretching

Dynamic stretching means pulling more or less brusquely on a muscle using small, repetitive movements for 10 to 20 seconds. Dynamic stretching resembles plyometrics because it plays with the stretch–relax cycle (or the elasticity of the muscle). The goal of the small movements is to force the muscle to lengthen more than it would naturally.

★ **Advantages:** This is least likely to cause a decrease in performance when done before a workout, so long as you do not tear a muscle. Be extremely careful when doing this type of stretching.

★ **Disadvantages:** Dynamic stretching is the most likely to cause a muscle tear. Generally people do 3 to 5 nonstop circuits of stretches. So the only thing you as a fighter need to do is determine which muscles you want to stretch depending on your fighting techniques. To help you in this task, see our book *Delavier's Stretching Anatomy.*

### BREATHING WHILE STRETCHING

Holding your breath during a stretch stiffens the muscle. When you are stretching, you need to relax your body. Inhale calmly and deeply to make the muscle lose as much of its resistance as possible. Synchronize your breath with the stretch; exhale during the most intense part of the stretch.

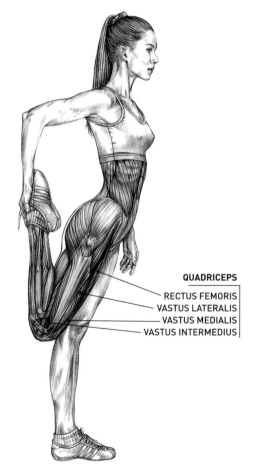

QUADRICEPS
RECTUS FEMORIS
VASTUS LATERALIS
VASTUS MEDIALIS
VASTUS INTERMEDIUS

**STRETCHING THE QUADRICEPS**

# TECHNIQUES FOR RECOVERY AND INJURY PREVENTION

The risk of injury in combat sports is especially high. Free fighting is no exception: There are an estimated 3 injuries in every 10 fights (Bledsoe et al., 2006, *Journal of Sports Science and Medicine*, 136-42). Injuries can also occur during strength training, and you do not want to add those to injuries suffered in the ring. To prevent injury, do the following:

→ Learn to warm up well before any exercise.
→ Do everything possible to accelerate recovery between workouts.

## WARM-UP

Think of the body as a car. If you accelerate quickly when the engine is cold, the car's speed will not increase much and you could damage the mechanical parts. However, when the engine is warm, a small acceleration will quickly increase the speed. In the same way, your muscles, tendons, and joints function optimally only at a certain temperature. It is imperative that you warm up before any kind of exercise for these reasons:

→ Guard against injury.
→ Optimize your performance.
→ Prepare yourself mentally for the effort to come.

You should always do 1 or 2 light warm-up sets before lifting heavy weights. These warm-up sets are not as intense, so you will not include them in the total number of sets you do in a workout.

### ♦ ADJUSTING YOUR WARM-UP
The amount of time you need to warm up can vary depending on the season and the time of day. In the winter, or early in the morning, your body is colder than in the summer or the afternoon, so you should add 1 or 2 sets to your warm-up. By compensating for the difference in temperature, you can eliminate any difference in performance. Since you should not shorten the rest of your workout, your total workout time will be a bit longer.

### ⚠ WARNING!

Many beginners think that they do not need to warm up. They think they can just start by lifting heavy weights because they do not want to waste time warming up. But skipping a warm-up will automatically result in pain later on, and that will restrict your fighting activities. A good preworkout warm-up protects against future aches and pains. Furthermore, it is also an immediate factor in improving performance.

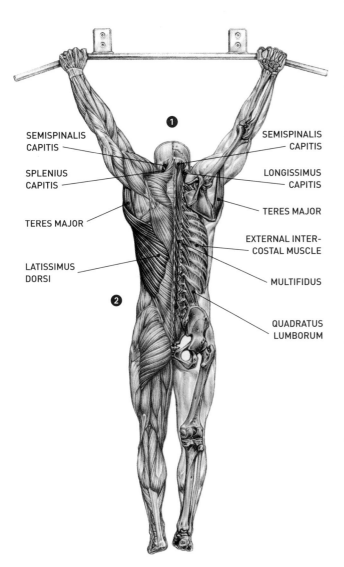

SEMISPINALIS CAPITIS

SPLENIUS CAPITIS

TERES MAJOR

LATISSIMUS DORSI

SEMISPINALIS CAPITIS

LONGISSIMUS CAPITIS

TERES MAJOR

EXTERNAL INTER-COSTAL MUSCLE

MULTIFIDUS

QUADRATUS LUMBORUM

❶ Tilt your head forward and try to touch your chin to your chest.

❷ Slowly relax your back and feel the stretch in the small intervertebral muscles.

Just as it is essential to warm up, it is equally important to relax the muscles at the end of a workout. Strength training tends to compress the spine and the joints, so you need to decompress them.

Decompression techniques were developed for professional American football teams. American football is a sport with rampant joint trauma. To get an injured player back on his feet quickly, the painful joint is decompressed.

As a way to prevent injuries, decompression is a technique that you should use as soon as possible after a workout. Joint traction removes some of the pressure exerted on the joint, which promotes blood flow and recovery. However, this does not mean pulling so hard that you injure your limb. Use natural joint traction by using gravity rather than by applying outside force or pulling on a joint.

To accelerate recovery in the lower back, decompress your spine by hanging from a pull-up bar for at least 30 seconds. You should feel your spine lengthening just from the effects of your body weight. If, however, your spine remains tight, this means your lumbar muscles are still experiencing a spasm. Relaxing them is something you will learn to do over time.

When you hang from a pull-up bar, you are not just stretching your spine; your wrists, elbows, and shoulders are also decompressed and experience the same regenerative benefits. Another decompression technique is to hang by your feet from a pull-up bar. Inversion, by placing your head down low and your feet up high, stretches the spine and prevents lower back pain. Hanging by the feet also decompresses the ankles, knees, and hips, which puts your recovery time ahead of schedule. Lymphatic circulation is accelerated because of natural drainage, and this is particularly noticeable after a workout.

The first few times that you have your head down low, it can be uncomfortable. You might feel that your face and your eyes are filling with blood. These symptoms are similar to those experienced by astronauts during their first days in space.

Common sense tells you that if this position is too uncomfortable, then you should avoid it. But during a fight on the ground, your opponent could hold your legs in the air and your head might be down low. If this position makes you disoriented, then you will lose the fight. Your future opponents will know exactly how to beat you as well. Therefore, it is smart to practice this so that you will be able to tolerate having your head low, especially when you are tired and out of breath.

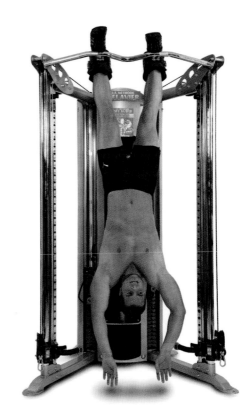

Inversion decompresses the spine and improves lymphatic circulation.

The best way to prepare for this inverted position is to practice using gravity boots regularly.

## REGENERATIVE MASSAGE USING A FOAM ROLLER

The accumulation of muscle and tendon microtraumas stimulates the development of nonelastic fibers. These fibers create adhesions between different layers within the muscle. This makes the muscle less flexible and more fragile, and eventually the muscle will have difficulty contracting powerfully. In addition to causing pain, it will decrease your performance.

The goal of myofascial release massage is to break these adhesions, or at least make them more flexible, in order to restore flexibility, strength, and speed to the muscle. To do this, you can massage yourself using a foam roller or a hard foam tube instead of visiting a massage therapist.

When you lie on a foam roller, you use your body weight to break down the adhesions as you roll the various muscle groups over the tube. Though you might think of this as a gadget at first, you will quickly realize that this is a technique that

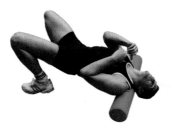

**1** Massaging the back, trapezius muscles, and neck

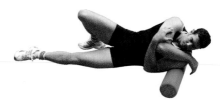

**2** Massaging the back of the shoulders and triceps muscles

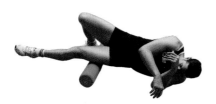

**3** Massaging the hamstrings and buttocks

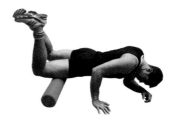

**4** Massaging the quadriceps

can actually be very painful. Fortunately, you control exactly how much pressure is applied on the tube, so you can be sure it will not hurt too much.

At first, you can also start out supporting some of your body weight on the floor with your hands and knees. This way, only the superficial layers of muscles are massaged, and it will not be as painful. The second time, you can work on the deeper layers by using your entire body weight. Similarly, the harder the roller is, the more effective the massage is (and the more painful it will be). A hard roller

that does not compress will help you better target specific muscle points.

You can massage yourself for 5 to 10 minutes on rest days. Focus on vulnerable areas like the shoulders and the lower back as well as around the knees and ankles. Between strength training sets, you can also massage yourself. Medical research has shown that using a foam roller facilitates recovery and thereby relieves fatigue (Healey et al., 2011, *Journal of Strength and Conditioning Research*, 25:S30-31).

## INJURY-CAUSING STRENGTH IMBALANCES

An increase in muscle strength is much more pronounced than an increase in joint strength. For example, compared to sedentary people, weightlifters have the following features:

→ Quadriceps are 26% stronger.
→ Hamstrings are only 11% stronger, which underscores the disparity in

strength between these two antagonistic muscles.
→ Knee cartilage is only 5% thicker (Gratzke et al., 2007, *American Journal of Sports Medicine*, 35(8):1346-53).

If you add to this the fact that, after a certain number of years of training, cartilage breaks down more than it thickens, then it is easy to understand the growing number of injuries.

#### ♦ CONCLUSION

An incomplete strength training program can result in strength imbalances. These imbalances predispose an athlete to various disabling problems. In this context, prevention is your best weapon. Be sure that you are developing the various antagonistic muscles equally. Your strength training program should strive to achieve balance between the following areas:

→ Front and back of the shoulders
→ Upper and lower trapezius muscles
→ Back and chest
→ Forearm flexors and extensors
→ Lumbar and abdominal muscles
→ Quadriceps and hamstrings

## CROSS-EDUCATION FOR RECOVERY FROM INJURY

If you are right-handed, your handwriting is best when you write with your right hand, and it probably does not look very good when you write with your left hand. The opposite is true for left-handed people. Nevertheless, you can still write with your nondominant hand, even though it is awkward. Yet no one ever taught you how to write with both hands. It is simply a partial transfer of the right hand's training to the left hand. This is called cross-education. This transfer phenomenon, coming solely from the nervous system, also exists in strength training. This means that if you work only your right arm, your left arm also gets stronger. This transfer represents about 10% to 15% of the gains realized on the side you are developing. That might seem like a small amount, but if you are injured and cannot train on one side, you should continue training on your good side. This will preserve the maximum amount of strength and it will be easier to start training those immobilized muscles again once the injury has healed.

## NUTRITIONAL APPROACH TO RECOVERY

This means using natural nutritional supplements to accelerate the recovery of muscles and joints. For example, high-level athletes with knee problems took either one or the other of the following each day for 28 days:

→ A placebo
→ 1.5 grams of glucosamine

Recovery of range of motion in the thigh was 40% faster with glucosamine than with placebo (Ostojic, et al., 2007, *Research in Sports Medicine*, 15(2):113-24).

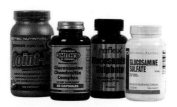

Some nutritional supplements can facilitate recovery.

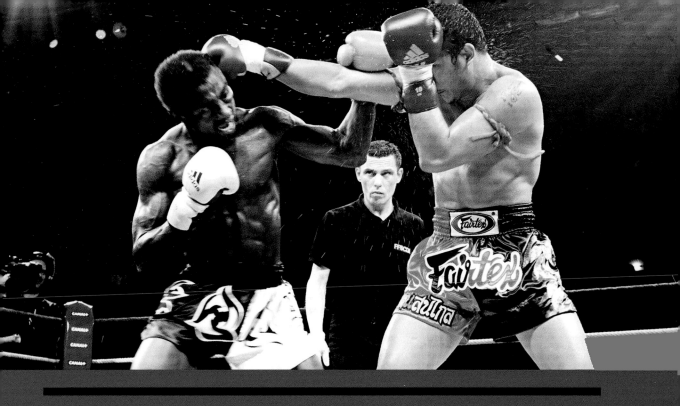

# STRENGTH TRAINING
# EXERCISES FOR FIGHTING

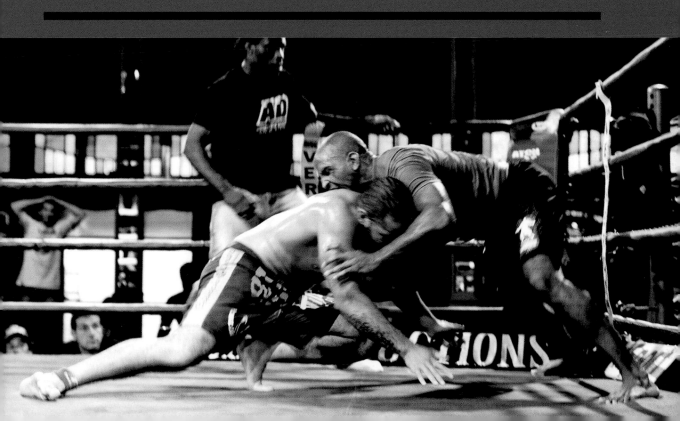

MOST STRENGTH TRAINING EXERCISES COME FROM BODYBUILDING, AND THE GOAL IN DOING THE EXERCISES IS TO ISOLATE A SPECIFIC MUSCLE OR GROUP OF MUSCLES. AS A FIGHTER, YOU DO NOT HAVE TO FOLLOW THIS NONFUNCTIONAL ISOLATION APPROACH. ON THE CONTRARY, YOU SHOULD USE EXERCISES THAT DIRECTLY IMPROVE YOUR FIGHTING MOVES, NOT JUST ONE OR TWO MUSCLES.

THE ONLY EXCEPTIONS TO THIS RULE ARE THE PASSIVE DEFENSIVE MUSCLES: NECK, TRA-PEZIUS, JAW, AND ABDOMINAL WALL.

YOU SHOULD ALSO BE AWARE THAT JUST BECAUSE YOU ARE DEVELOPING YOUR MUSCLES, IT DOES NOT MEAN YOU ARE NOT ALSO CREATING PROBLEMS AT THE SAME TIME, ESPECIALLY IN THE JOINTS. WE NOTE ANY INHERENT DANGER IN AN EXERCISE, IF IT EXISTS, SO AS TO MINIMIZE THE RISKS. YOU SHOULD ALSO CHOOSE EXERCISES THAT OFFER THE BEST COMPRO-MISE BETWEEN EFFECTIVENESS AND RISK, DEPENDING ON YOUR BODY TYPE.

# NECK, TRAPEZIUS, AND JAW

As a fighter, you not only throw punches, but you also get hit. This is why it is essen-tial to protect the vulnerable areas: your head and neck. If we take the example of a gorilla, it would be very difficult to choke him or knock him out because of his mas-sive neck and trapezius muscles. So he can serve as a model for fighters. A fighter has a special interest in developing the muscles in this area.

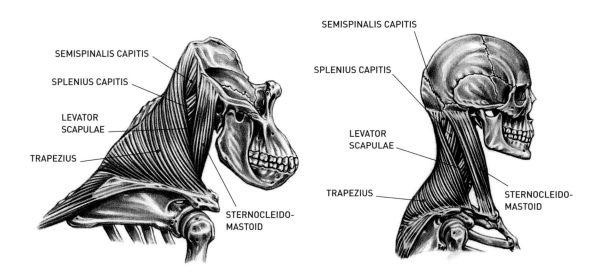

SEMISPINALIS CAPITIS
SPLENIUS CAPITIS
LEVATOR SCAPULAE
TRAPEZIUS
STERNOCLEIDO-MASTOID

SEMISPINALIS CAPITIS
SPLENIUS CAPITIS
LEVATOR SCAPULAE
TRAPEZIUS
STERNOCLEIDO-MASTOID

## Role of the Neck Muscles

The muscles in the neck have three roles:

★ **1.** They provide mobility in the neck.

★ **2.** Because of this great mobility, as well as the significant weight of the head, the cervical vertebrae take a lot of abuse during a fight. Therefore, the second role of the neck muscles is to protect the cervical vertebrae, especially in case of a hit. For this reason, working this part of the body is especially important for a fighter.

★ **3.** Visually, a large neck is always impressive. So the third role is to intimidate an opponent with your large neck.

## A Large, Vulnerable Area

In addition to being the weak link in a fight, the neck is frequently subject to injuries.

For example, 20% of wrestlers suffer from neck pain starting in their first year of activity.

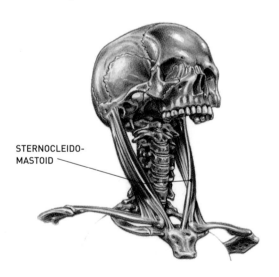

The sternocleidomastoid participates independently in the rotation of the head.

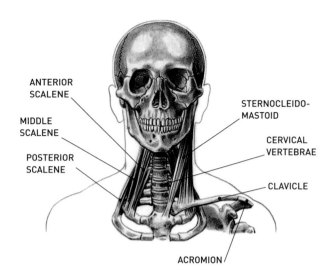

This figure climbs to 50% in the following years, because once a fighter is injured, the risk of developing a new lesion skyrockets. The incidence of neck pain also increases as a fighter ages.

There are two primary factors in the risk of a neck injury, and strength training can help you improve both of them.

★ **1.** Muscle weakness in the neck

★ **2.** Strength imbalances between different muscles in the neck

For people who have not been working out, extension strength is twice as high as flexion strength (Ylinen et al., 2003, *Journal of Strength and Conditioning Research*, 17:755-9). This imbalance persists even among fighters. Compared to sedentary people, the neck strength of high-level fighters is

→ 60% greater in extension,
→ 120% greater in flexion, and
→ 170% greater in rotation.

This imbalance is one risk factor for injury that you should be able to eliminate through focused training. In fact, when you fall on your back, it is important to have strong neck flexors so that you can

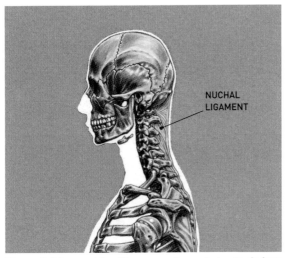

NUCHAL LIGAMENT

The nuchal ligament is a fibrous membrane that extends from the base of the skull to the bottom of the neck. It rigidifies and protects the neck by preventing movements that are so large that they could damage the spinal cord.

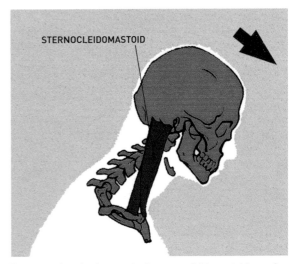

STERNOCLEIDOMASTOID

By contracting simultaneously, the sternocleidomastoid muscles thrust the head forward, as in a head butt.

pull your head forward powerfully. If the neck muscles are tight (the head stays backward), then the shock endured is similar to what you would experience in a car accident that causes whiplash.

So it is an excellent idea to strengthen the neck by endowing it with large muscles. To do this, unlike with other muscles, it will help to use some muscle hypertrophy techniques borrowed from bodybuilding.

## Muscle Qualities You Should Develop

The goal of powerful musculature is to minimize the stretching of numerous ligaments that hold the cervical vertebrae in place when the head is hit. For the neck, the main quality desired is isometric strength as well as the ability to absorb blows (negative strength). So you will do slow, or even static, work. You will also need endurance, because the risk of injury increases as you fatigue. This means you need to do a large number of sets so that you can repeat strength exercises on an already-tired muscle.

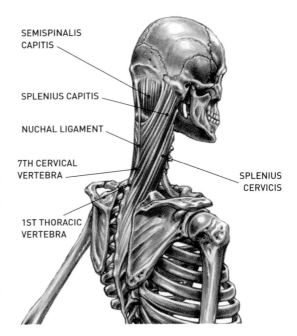

SEMISPINALIS CAPITIS

SPLENIUS CAPITIS

NUCHAL LIGAMENT

7TH CERVICAL VERTEBRA

1ST THORACIC VERTEBRA

SPLENIUS CERVICIS

**EXTENSOR MUSCLES OF THE NECK, THREE-QUARTER VIEW**

## Isolate to Develop a Muscle

Traditional strength training exercises work the neck very little; therefore, specific isolation exercises are required. A complete program for the neck should include exercises for the muscles in these areas:

→ Front of the neck (flexor muscles)
→ Back of the neck (extensor muscles)
→ Sides of the neck (rotator muscles)

Here we provide the exercises that are the least traumatic for each area of the neck. Only after several months of strengthening your neck using these exercises can you move on to wrestling exercises, which are much more dangerous, such as the bridge or any other perilous maneuver where you use your head as a support.

## ⚠ WARNING!

Since the cervical vertebrae are small, it is easy to hurt them. Strength training develops the neck muscles to protect the cervical spine during fights. But you must not lose sight of the fact that you can also injure your cervical vertebrae just by doing strength training exercises. For an athlete who is already injured, strength training can easily exacerbate an already painful condition. Strengthening the muscles should reduce the neck's vulnerability, not make it worse. To avoid efforts that are counterproductive to your goals, you must do neck exercises in a controlled manner and in long sets (20 to 30 repetitions). This will help prevent damage to your cervical vertebrae.

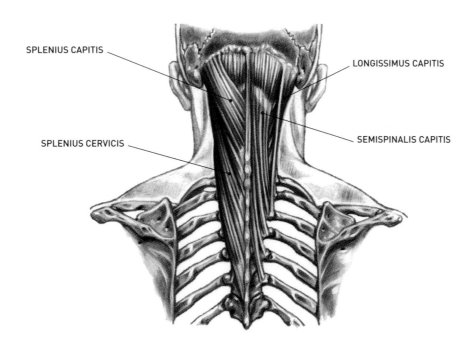

SPLENIUS CAPITIS

LONGISSIMUS CAPITIS

SPLENIUS CERVICIS

SEMISPINALIS CAPITIS

**EXTENSOR MUSCLES OF THE NECK, BACK VIEW**

## NECK FLEXION

*This is an isolation exercise for the muscles in the front of the neck. It is the most important exercise you can do to protect the cervical vertebrae if you fall on your back.*

**Stand or kneel, bring your fists together, and place them under your chin ❶. Use your neck to push on your fists and bring your head down as far down as you can ❷. Hold this position for 5 seconds as you squeeze the muscles as hard as you can.**

**Slowly push your head back up with your fists, and resist the movement with your neck.**

### HELPFUL HINTS

Do not bring your head up too high in the stretched position. It is best if your chin does not go too far past the point where it is parallel to the floor.

### VARIATIONS

❹ If you already have neck pain, you can do this exercise isometrically to avoid any movement. Place your fists between your chest and neck. Squeeze your neck muscles as

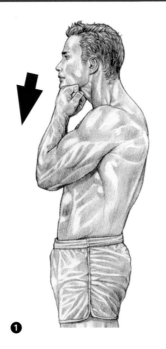

❶

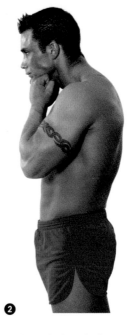

❷

hard as possible. Hold the position for at least 10 seconds and then relax for a few seconds. Repeat until fatigued.
❸ Instead of keeping your head straight, turn it 45 degrees to the right for 1 set, and then do another set with your head turned to the left.
❹ To make this exercise more difficult, lie on your back on a bench so that your head hangs off the bench. Put a weight plate on your chest and put a towel on top of it so your head will not touch the weight. Tilt your head back

and then bring it forward toward the weight.
❹ To add resistance, you can place a strap around your head and attach it to a

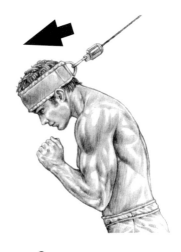

❹ **USING A HIGH PULLEY**

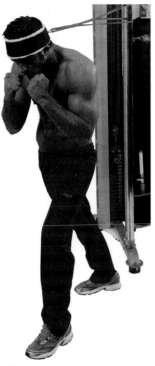

high pulley or to an elastic band.

❺ There are machines that simulate neck flexion exercises.

## ADVANTAGES

Using your hands works the neck while decompressing the cervical vertebrae, which is a good thing.

## DISADVANTAGES

Since the resistance is manual, it is hard to gauge the level of resistance you are placing on your muscles. For this reason, it is hard to know how much strength you are gaining.

Using actual weights as resistance eliminates this difficulty but is also more traumatic for your cervical vertebrae than using manual resistance.

## ⚠ RISKS

To avoid putting pressure on your cervical vertebrae, be careful not to lift your head too high.

**Ⓓ USING AN ELASTIC BAND**

# NECK EXTENSION

*This is an isolation exercise for the muscles at the back of the neck. These muscles (splenius) give a boxer's neck its characteristic shape. They help you to avoid getting knocked out when you are hit in the head.*

**Stand or kneel, intertwine your fingers, and put your hands behind the upper part of your head ❶.**

**Use the strength in your neck to push your hands backward as far as possible ❷.**

**Hold this position for 5 seconds and squeeze your**

**muscles as hard as you can. Slowly bring your head forward using your hands as you resist with your neck.**

## HELPFUL HINTS

Do not push your head too far down in the stretched position. It is best if your chin does not go much past the point where it is parallel to the floor.

## NOTES

You can do neck extensions and neck flexion exercises in a super-set with no breaks in between.

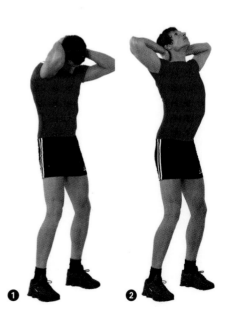

## VARIATIONS

**Ⓐ** To avoid all movement if your neck is already sore, you can do this exercise statically. Lie on a bed with your back flat and then push your head down as far as possible into the mattress. Hold that position for at least 10 seconds and then relax for a few seconds. Repeat until fatigued.

**Ⓑ** You can do the same exercise standing with your back against a wall.

**Ⓒ** Instead of keeping your head straight, turn it 45 degrees to the right for 1 set, and then do another set with your head turned to the left.

**Ⓓ** Instead of using your hands, you can place a towel or an elastic band behind your head for resistance.

**Ⓔ** To make this exercise more difficult, lie facedown on a bench so that your head hangs off the bench. Put a towel on your head and then put a weight plate on the towel so your head does not touch the weight. Lean your head toward the floor and then bring it back up.

**Ⓕ** To add resistance, you can place a strap around your head and attach it to a pulley or an elastic band.

**Ⓖ** There are machines that simulate neck extension exercises.

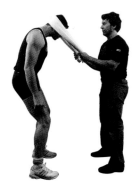

**Ⓓ USING A TOWEL HELD BY A PARTNER**

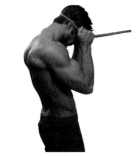

**Ⓓ USING AN ELASTIC BAND**

## ADVANTAGES

Using your hands or an elastic band works the neck without compressing the cervical spine, as can happen when you do weighted variations or use a machine.

## DISADVANTAGES

Moving the neck in this way can cause vertigo. This is why you must do the exercise very slowly and under continuous tension. If you have vertigo, try the exercise with your eyes closed to see if that resolves the problem.

### ⚠ RISKS

Never apply pressure toward the floor with your hands, because this could compress the cervical vertebrae.

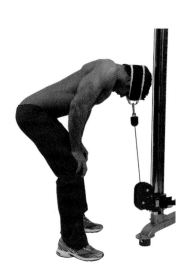

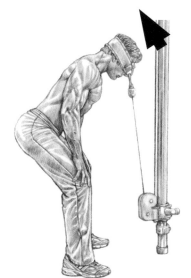

**Ⓕ USING A PULLEY**

*This is an isolation exercise for the muscles on the side of the neck.*

**Stand or kneel, and put the palm of your right hand above your right ear ❶. Use your neck to push your hand as far as possible toward the right ❷. Hold this position for at least 5 seconds and squeeze the muscles as hard as you can. Then slowly push your head back toward the starting position as you resist with your neck. Once you have worked the right side, move immediately to the left side.**

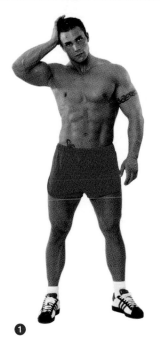

❶

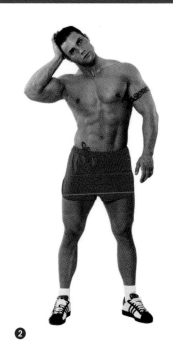

❷

### HELPFUL HINTS

Do not overwork the range of motion in your neck, especially in the lengthened position. Whether you are in the lengthened or contracted position, do not bend your head too far.

### NOTES

Maintain continuous tension and work slowly in an almost isometric fashion.

### VARIATIONS

❹ If your neck is already sore, you can do this exercise statically to avoid all movement.
❸ To add resistance, you can place a strap around your head and attach it to a pulley or an elastic band.
❻ Instead of pushing with your hand, you can use your hand to pull (see page 64).
❼ To make this exercise more difficult, lie on your side so that you can use the weight of your head as resistance. Once this variation becomes too easy, add a small weight plate on top of the ear that is facing the ceiling.

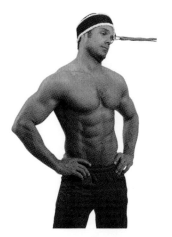

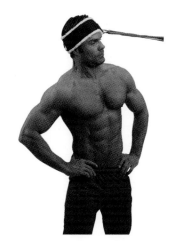

**❸ USING AN ELASTIC BAND**

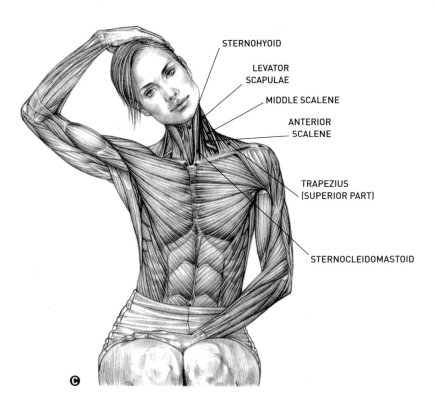

STERNOHYOID

LEVATOR SCAPULAE

MIDDLE SCALENE

ANTERIOR SCALENE

TRAPEZIUS (SUPERIOR PART)

STERNOCLEIDOMASTOID

Ⓒ

## ADVANTAGES

This exercise works the protective muscles of the neck, which are normally difficult to isolate.

## DISADVANTAGES

Any sudden movement could injure the cervical spine. Stay focused throughout this exercise.

## ⚠ RISKS

Lateral work is without a doubt the most dangerous kind of exercise for the neck. Use only a very small range of motion.

## STRENGTHENING THE JAW

If the slightest punch to your chin could dislocate your jaw, then you need to strengthen the muscles that rigidify the temporomandibular joint. Jaw dislocations are debilitating and painful, but you can prevent them by strengthening the supporting muscles. You can do this by chewing several pieces of gum at the same time. However, you should not open your mouth too wide because you could actually train your jaw to dislocate rather than to remain rigid. You can also practice the opposite movement to strengthen the antagonistic muscles. To do this, open your mouth while holding both fists under your jaw for resistance.

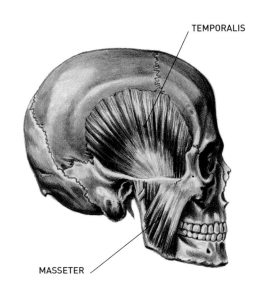

TEMPORALIS

MASSETER

The trapezius muscles have three purposes:

★ **1.** In addition to the strength they provide, the trapezius muscles protect the neck. Aesthetically, large trapezius muscles can hide your neck.

★ **2.** The combination of large trapezius muscles and a thick neck is ideal for intimidating opponents.

★ **3.** The lower trapezius stabilizes and protects the shoulder joint. A strength imbalance between the upper and lower trapezius promotes deltoid injuries. You can strengthen this region through rowing (see page 123).

## Role of Trapezius Muscles

The trapezius muscles are divided into three parts:

★ **1.** The upper part raises the shoulders. This is the part that fighters are most interested in developing.

★ **2.** The lower part performs the task opposite the upper part by lowering the shoulders.

★ **3.** The middle part brings the shoulder blades together.

**PARTS OF THE TRAPEZIUS**

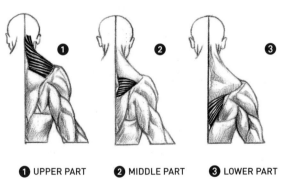

**❶** UPPER PART  **❷** MIDDLE PART  **❸** LOWER PART

TRAPEZIUS

CLAVICLE

ACROMION

SCAPULAR SPINE

SCAPULA

RIB

THORACIC VERTEBRAE

## SHRUG

*This is an isolation exercise for the upper trapezius.*

**Stand with your arms by your sides and grab either a long bar, or two dumbbells, or two kettlebells ❶. Or, use a shrug machine.**

**Bring your shoulders up as high as possible, as if you were trying to touch your trapezius muscles to your ears ❷. Hold the contracted position for 1 second before lowering your shoulders.**

**You should stretch as far as you can without hearing any popping noises in your neck (noises indicate that the cervical vertebrae are moving slightly).**

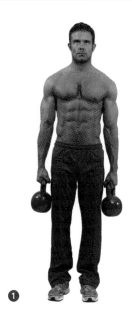

❶

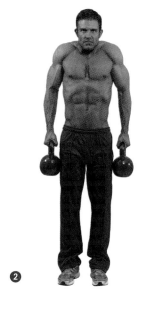

❷

### HELPFUL HINTS

Do not bend your arms at the beginning of the movement. However, once your shoulders are up, you can pull lightly with your biceps to raise your shoulders just a bit higher ❸.

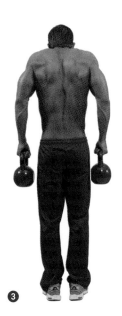

❸

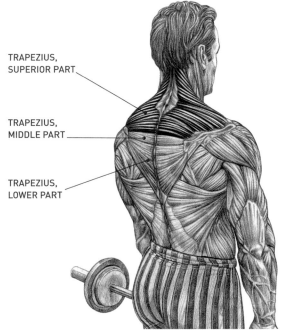

TRAPEZIUS, SUPERIOR PART

TRAPEZIUS, MIDDLE PART

TRAPEZIUS, LOWER PART

Ⓑ **WITH A LONG BAR IN FRONT OF THE BODY, USING A PRONATED GRIP**

## VARIATIONS

**Ⓐ** Using dumbbells: You can hold them in front of or behind your body as well as at your sides in order to change the angle of focus on your trapezius muscles.

**Ⓑ** Using a long bar: You can hold your hands in front of your body (pronated grip) or behind you (pronated or supinated grip).

**Ⓒ** Using a machine or a bar: You can adjust the width of your hands to work your trapezius muscles from unusual angles.

**Ⓓ** To reduce the dangling of a bar, you can also do shrugs inside a squat rack with or without hands.

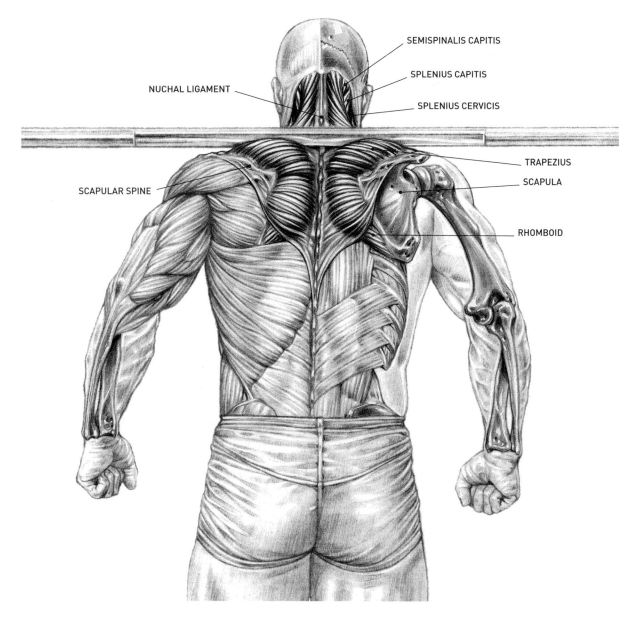

SEMISPINALIS CAPITIS

SPLENIUS CAPITIS

NUCHAL LIGAMENT

SPLENIUS CERVICIS

TRAPEZIUS

SCAPULA

SCAPULAR SPINE

RHOMBOID

**Ⓓ DELAVIER'S SHRUG IN A SQUAT RACK USING NO HANDS**

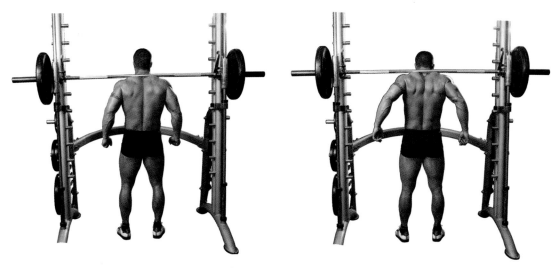

**D IN A SQUAT RACK USING NO HANDS**

The difference between a classic shrug and Delavier's shrug is that Delavier's shrug better targets the upper fibers of the trapezius that insert on the scapular spine. The classic shrug targets the upper fibers that insert on the clavicle.

## ADVANTAGES

This exercise works the trapezius muscles directly. The only interference comes from your hands, which may have trouble maintaining their grip during a very heavy set. Using a belt (from judo, for instance) will solve this problem **① ② ③**.

## DISADVANTAGES

Repeated contractions of the upper trapezius muscles can cause headaches because of the muscles' proximity to the cervical spine. So you should introduce this exercise carefully.

## ⚠ RISKS

Since it is possible to lift very heavy weights during this exercise, you could compress your lumbar vertebrae. Be careful not to hurt your back when lifting heavy weights.

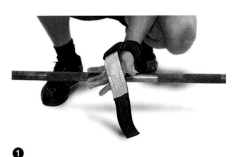

**①**

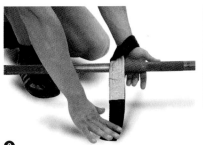

**②**

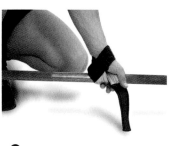

**③**

Using a belt or strap to strengthen your hand grip

# ABDOMINAL WALL

In fighting, more than in any other sport, the demands placed on the abdomen are enormous:

→ It must be well supported so that it protects your internal organs when you get hit.
→ It needs to function as a solid link between your thighs and torso.
→ It must have strength and endurance to increase the effectiveness of your strikes, all while remaining supple and extremely mobile so you can dodge attacks despite the continual abuse the abdomen takes.

Because of this complexity, you should work your abdominal wall from several angles. Do not neglect a single angle if you want to be at your best during a fight.

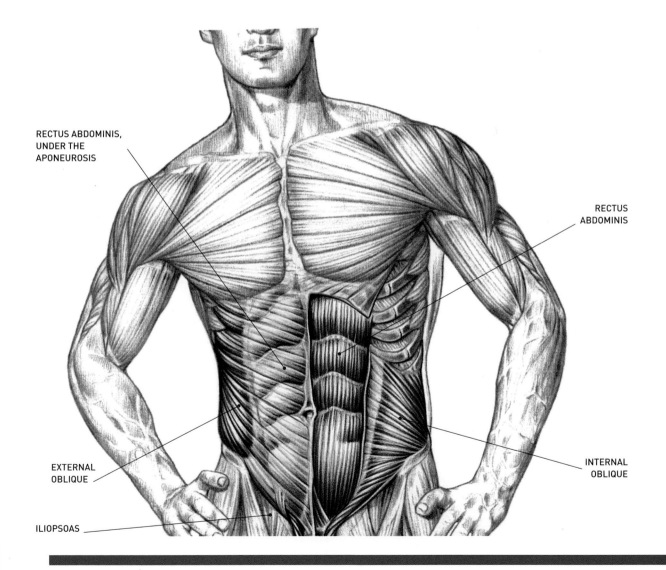

RECTUS ABDOMINIS, UNDER THE APONEUROSIS

RECTUS ABDOMINIS

EXTERNAL OBLIQUE

INTERNAL OBLIQUE

ILIOPSOAS

In quadrupeds, the muscles of the abdominal wall passively support the internal organs like a hammock and generally play a relatively limited active role in locomotion.

Because humans walk on two legs, the muscles in the abdominal wall are considerably stronger than the abdominal muscles of quadrupeds. In the vertical position, they stabilize the pelvis with the torso, preventing the torso from swinging too much while walking or running. Abdominal muscles have become powerful restraining muscles that actively support the internal organs.

❶ RECTUS ABDOMINIS
❷ EXTERNAL OBLIQUE
❸ INTERNAL OBLIQUE
❹ TRANSVERSUS ABDOMINIS

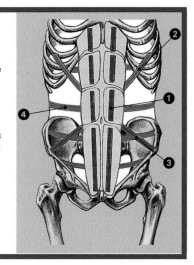

# SIT-UP

*This is an isolation exercise for the entire abdominal wall and the hip flexors.*

### WHY FIGHTERS SHOULD DO IT

★ To strengthen the entire abdominal wall to protect the internal organs

★ To develop the hip flexors, which are indispensable when doing powerful kicks with the feet or knees (see sections starting on page 94)

**Lie on your back with your legs bent and your feet flat on the floor. Tuck your feet under a machine or a wall bar, or have a partner hold them. Place your hands by your ears ❶.**

**Lift your shoulders so that your torso comes off the floor. You should curl**

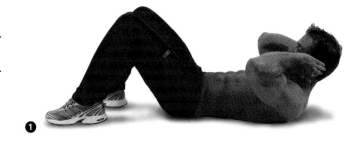

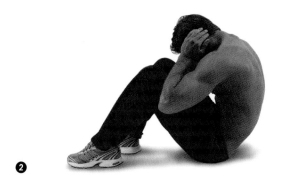

**up quickly until your torso touches your thighs ❷.**

**Return to the starting position and begin again,** always without any abrupt movements.

## HELPFUL HINTS

The placement of your hands changes the difficulty of this exercise. To move from the most difficult to the easiest variation, begin doing sit-ups with your arms held straight out behind you ❸. When you get tired, put your hands on your shoulders so you can do a few more repetitions.

End by giving your arms momentum as you do shadow boxing movements.

## NOTES

Exhale as you contract your abdomen and inhale as you lower your torso to the floor.

## VARIATIONS

Ⓐ To increase the resistance, you can hold a weight plate behind your head or a dumbbell on your chest.

Ⓑ Instead of lying on the floor, you can do sit-ups on an inclined ab bench that holds your feet. The higher you place your feet, the more difficult the exercise becomes.

Ⓒ Lie on a fitness ball or a BOSU ball to increase the range of motion in the exercise.

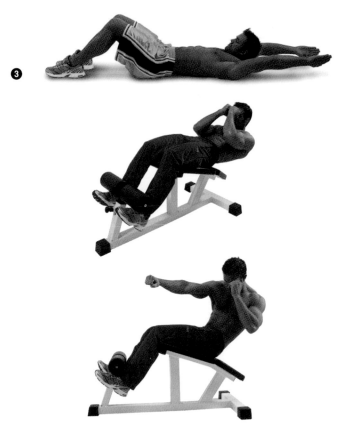

❸

Ⓑ Performing a sit-up on an ab bench

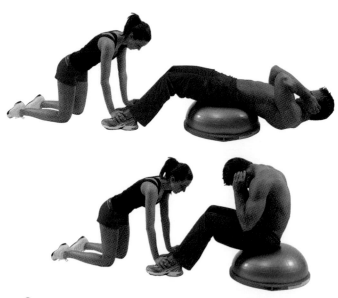

Ⓒ Performing a sit-up on a BOSU ball with a partner holding the feet

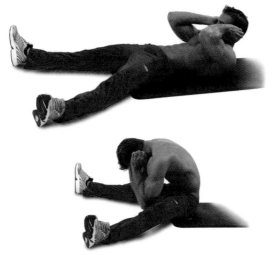

**E** Move from lying on your back on the floor to a standing position by doing a sit-up and then using one arm to help you get up. Over time, try to use the arm less and less.

Each time, stand up as quickly as you can so that you get used to jumping back up into a fighting stance.

**D** Performing a sit-up with the legs almost straight

**D** Rather than bend your legs to 90 degrees, some people prefer to keep them nearly straight to accentuate the role of the hip flexors.

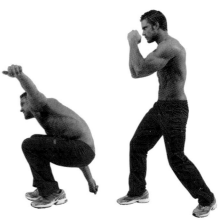

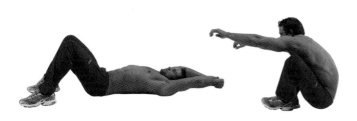

**E** Performing a sit-up to the standing position

### ADVANTAGES
Sit-ups are the most complete exercise for the abdominal wall and hip flexors.

### DISADVANTAGES
As the tension generated by the hip flexors increases, the lumbar spine suffers. If you have even the slightest pain in your discs, you should not do this exercise.

### ⚠ RISKS
Do not arch backward. On the contrary, round your back forward as much as you can to protect your spinal column.

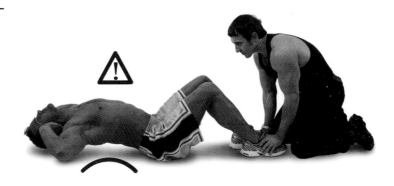

*This isolation exercise works the entire abdominal wall, especially the upper rectus abdominis muscle.*

## WHY FIGHTERS SHOULD DO IT

★ To be able to hold an opponent against the floor or the cage

★ To increase overall power in hand-to-hand fighting

**Stand with a high pulley behind you. Grab the cable rope attachment ❶. Quickly bend your torso forward as if you were getting ready to hit an opponent during a hand-to-hand fight ❷. Go down about 20 inches before returning to the starting position.**

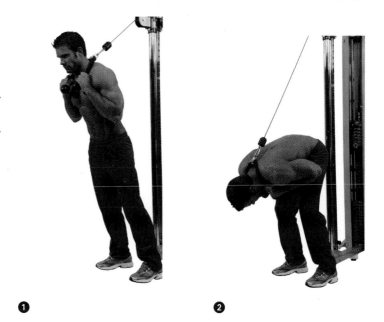

❶   ❷

## VARIATIONS

❹ Kneel with a high pulley behind you. You can use a triceps strap or bar. Curl your torso forward as if you were trying to pin an opponent on the ground. Hold the contracted position for 10 seconds before returning to the starting position.

❸ Lie on your back on the floor and use a low pulley that is placed behind your head. Grab the handle and keep the cord between your neck

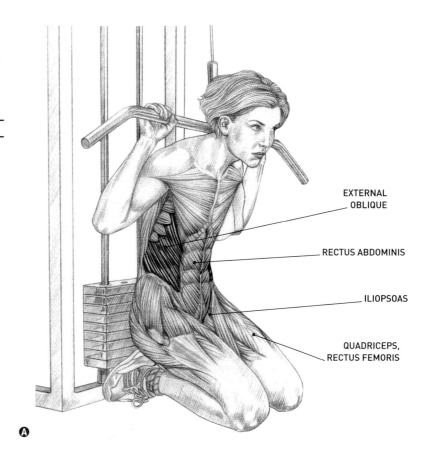

EXTERNAL OBLIQUE

RECTUS ABDOMINIS

ILIOPSOAS

QUADRICEPS, RECTUS FEMORIS

❹

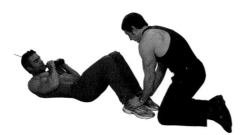 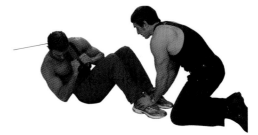

**B** Performing the exercise while lying down

and left shoulder. Pull diagonally as if you were trying to get out from under an opponent who is pinning you to the ground. Lift the left side of your torso at least 10 inches (25 cm) before lowering to the starting position. After you have done a set of cord twists on the left, do the same exercise with the cord on the right side of your body.

## HELPFUL HINTS

In all three versions of the exercise, keep your back slightly curved forward. Never arch backward!

## ADVANTAGES

The pulley helps you adjust the resistance in the exercise perfectly. The abdominal muscles are worked very differently depending on the technique you choose (plyometric in the primary exercise and variation **B**; isometric in variation **A**).

## DISADVANTAGES

Beyond a certain weight, it becomes difficult to stay firmly anchored on the floor and to control the trajectory of your torso precisely as you come back up. But you will have to deal with these issues during a fight.

## ⚠ RISKS

If the weight is controlling the movement, then in the best case your movements could be random. In the worst case, you could hurt yourself.

---

# TWISTING CRUNCH

*This isolation exercise targets the internal and external obliques as well as the rectus abdominis.*

## WHY FIGHTERS SHOULD DO IT

★ To make punches stronger by increasing the activation of the abdominal muscles
★ To get stronger so that you can get out of a hold

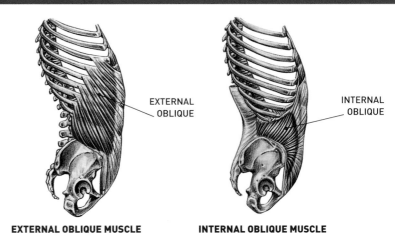

EXTERNAL OBLIQUE

INTERNAL OBLIQUE

**EXTERNAL OBLIQUE MUSCLE**          **INTERNAL OBLIQUE MUSCLE**

more easily when you are pinned on your back.

**Lie on your back with your legs bent and your feet tucked under a machine or a wall bar or held by a partner ❶. Place your hands near your ears or on a straight bar. Lift your right shoulder and bring your right elbow toward your left knee ❷ so that you twist to the left. Then twist to the right during the next repetition.**

## VARIATIONS

❹ To make this exercise harder, use an inclined ab bench instead of lying on the floor. You can make the exercise even more difficult by adding a weight.

❽ Lie on a stability ball or BOSU ball to increase the range of motion in the exercise.

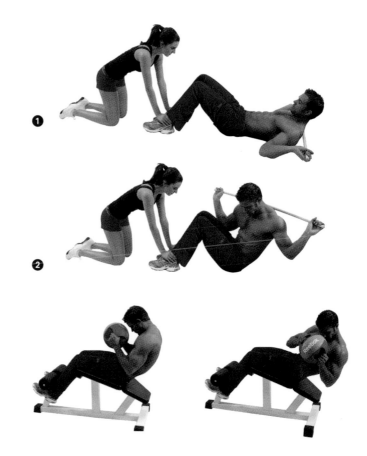

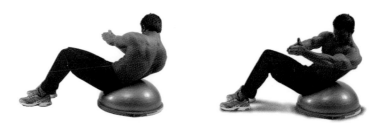

🅐 PERFORMING THE EXERCISE ON AN AB BENCH WITH A MEDICINE BALL

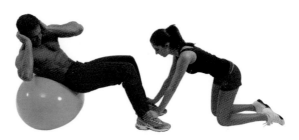

🅑 PERFORMING THE EXERCISE ON A BOSU BALL

🅑 PERFORMING THE EXERCISE ON A STABILITY BALL
WITH YOUR FEET HELD BY A PARTNER

◉ Instead of using your torso as a source of resistance, you can do this exercise using a pulley or an elastic band. With this variation, you can alter the direction of force by placing the pulley or the elastic band at a different height.

## ADVANTAGES

Twisting crunches are excellent training for fighters.

## DISADVANTAGES

Since you have to first work one side and then the other, you will end up spending a lot of time on this exercise.

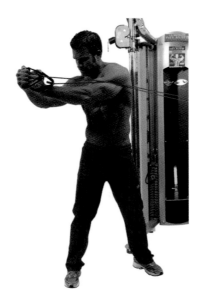

◉ **USING AN ELASTIC BAND**

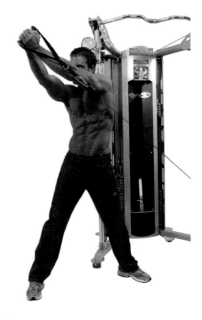

◉ **USING A PULLEY**

**⚠ RISKS**

To avoid injuring your discs, be careful of two things:

→ Do not twist farther than 10 inches (~25 cm).
→ Do not arch backward.

## IMPORTANCE OF TWISTING CRUNCHES IN A FIGHT

Many blows and strikes begin with a torso rotation. For example, when you throw a punch, you first rotate your torso backward as a kind of wind-up. It is very important to focus on the muscles responsible for these rotations so that you can do the following:

→ Rotate powerfully and thus increase the impact of your strikes.
→ Increase your ability to escape or flip an opponent over on the ground.
→ Prevent muscle injuries, which are quite common in this relatively fragile area.

You should do these rotations from both ends by using the following:

→ Your torso (which twists while your thighs remain stationary)
→ Your thighs (which twist while your torso remains stationary)

These are the two cases that you experience in a fight. The first happens while you are standing up and, occasionally, on the ground as you try to use your torso to turn over. The second happens when your back is on the ground as you gather momentum with your legs to flip your opponent over.

*This isolation exercise works the obliques.*

### WHY FIGHTERS SHOULD DO IT

★ To become accustomed to escaping from an opponent or flipping him over with your legs when you are on your back and pinned to the ground

Hang from a pull-up bar using an overhand grip (thumbs facing each other) with your hands slightly more than shoulder-width apart. Keep your legs straight and bring your feet up as high as you can toward the ceiling ❶.

Using your obliques, swing your legs to the right ❷. Do not rotate more than 90 degrees before coming back up. Then do a rotation to the left ❸.

### VARIATIONS

Ⓐ You can keep your legs straight so the exercise will be much more difficult, or you can bring your calves up to your thighs to make it easier.

Ⓑ If this exercise is too difficult on the pull-up bar, you can do it while lying on your back on the floor. You can stabilize your body by holding on to something with your hands.

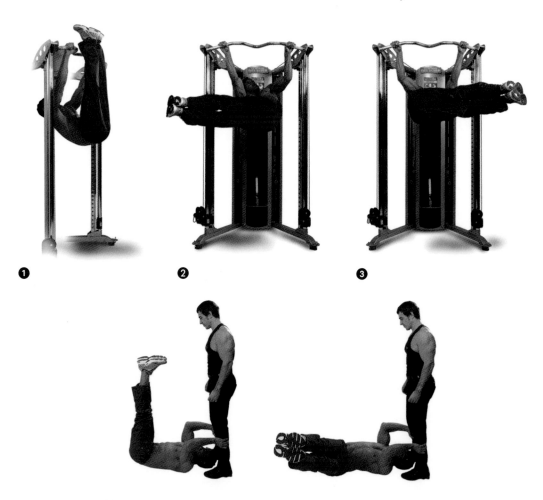

❶     ❷     ❸

Ⓑ PERFORMING THE EXERCISE WHILE HOLDING ON TO A PARTNER'S ANKLES

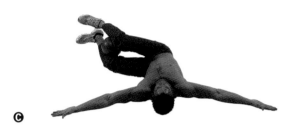

**⊙** When this exercise becomes too easy, try holding a medicine ball between your thighs. This will make the exercise harder and force you to work your adductors as if you were squeezing an opponent's torso in order to flip him with your legs.

**⊙**

### ADVANTAGES

In addition to the obliques, your arms and thighs provide an intense effort to stabilize your body, and this involves numerous muscles working together.

### DISADVANTAGES

Do not exaggerate the twisting motion.

### ⚠ RISKS

If you have back problems, you should not do this exercise.

## PLANK

*This isolation exercise works the entire abdominal wall isometrically.*

### WHY FIGHTERS SHOULD DO IT

★ To strengthen the abdominal wall and increase your static muscular endurance

Lie on the floor facedown, and support yourself on your elbows and toes (push-up position). Keep your body as straight as possible, and hold this static position for at least 30 seconds **❶**.

### HELPFUL HINTS

If you have trouble putting your palms on the floor, make fists and put your hands in a neutral position (with only the pinkies touching the floor). If the weight of your head becomes too uncomfortable, bend your neck forward so your head rests on your hands. A yoga mat will help prevent discomfort in your forearms.

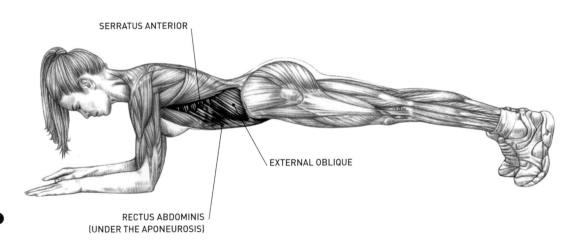

SERRATUS ANTERIOR

EXTERNAL OBLIQUE

**❶**

RECTUS ABDOMINIS
(UNDER THE APONEUROSIS)

## VARIATIONS

**Ⓐ** To increase the difficulty of this exercise, a partner can place a weight plate on your lower back or sit on you. In this case, be very careful not to arch your back.

**Ⓑ** If you do this exercise in a side position, you can focus the work on your obliques. If this variation is too difficult at first, put your free hand on the floor for support.

## ADVANTAGES

This stabilization exercise requires no equipment or material, and you can do it in very little time. Among fighters, it could become a friendly competition to see who can hold the position the longest.

## DISADVANTAGES

For the reasons mentioned at the beginning of this section, static work should never be the only way in which you work the abdominal wall.

## ⚠ RISKS

If you arch your back, you could pinch your discs. Even though holding your breath makes this exercise easier, you should not hold your breath! If you feel like your breathing is affected, exhale using tiny breaths.

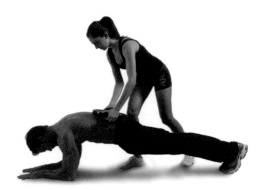

**Ⓐ USING A WEIGHT**

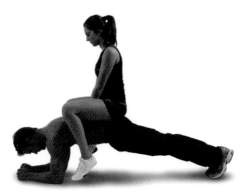

**Ⓐ WITH A PARTNER ON THE BACK**

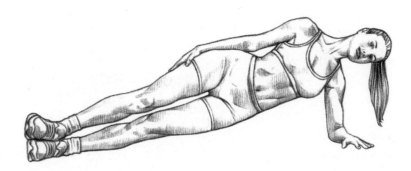

**Ⓑ**

# PUNCHES AND ELBOW STRIKES

Punches recruit almost all the muscles in the body. In addition to technique, the power in a punch depends on general muscle power as well as the coordination between muscle groups (thighs, torso rotation, and arms).

Of this trio of technique, power, and coordination, the following exercises focus on improving power and coordination.

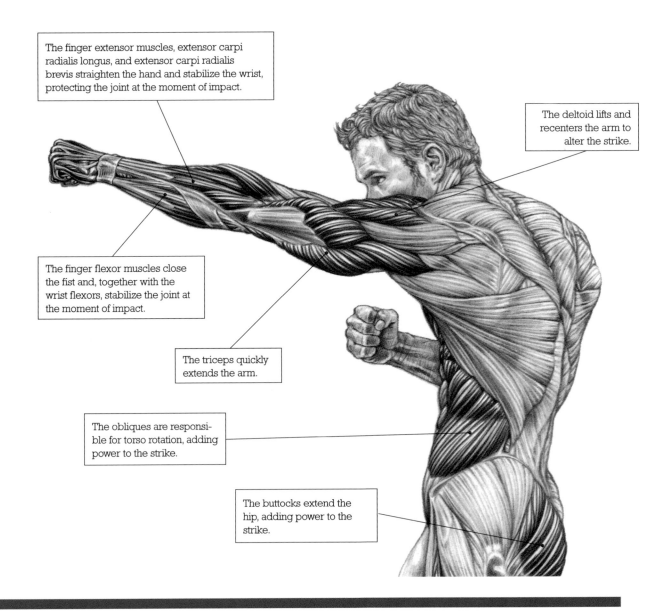

The finger extensor muscles, extensor carpi radialis longus, and extensor carpi radialis brevis straighten the hand and stabilize the wrist, protecting the joint at the moment of impact.

The deltoid lifts and recenters the arm to alter the strike.

The finger flexor muscles close the fist and, together with the wrist flexors, stabilize the joint at the moment of impact.

The triceps quickly extends the arm.

The obliques are responsible for torso rotation, adding power to the strike.

The buttocks extend the hip, adding power to the strike.

## NARROW-GRIP BENCH PRESS

*This is a compound exercise for the triceps, chest, and shoulders.*

### WHY FIGHTERS SHOULD DO IT

★ To strengthen all the muscles of the upper body, especially those that make punches and hammer fist strikes more powerful

★ To get stronger so you can push an opponent off of you when you are on your back

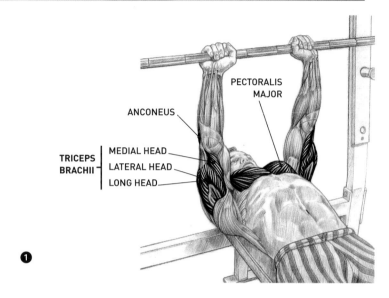

PECTORALIS MAJOR

ANCONEUS

TRICEPS BRACHII
— MEDIAL HEAD
— LATERAL HEAD
— LONG HEAD

❶

**Lie on a bench made for bench presses or in a squat rack. Use a pronated grip (thumbs facing each other) and grab the bar with your hands about as wide as you normally punch ❶. If you use a wider grip, you will get stronger, of course, but the muscle work will not correlate with the strikes you throw in a fight (since you rarely punch toward the outside). Lower the bar to your chest and then lift it up powerfully to straighten your arms.**

### HELPFUL HINTS

The narrower your grip and the farther out you place your elbows, the more you will work your triceps.

### VARIATIONS

Ⓐ Instead of doing repetitions nonstop, pause for a moment at the bottom of the exercise, resting the bar on the lower safeties in a stop-and-go style. Pause for at least 3 seconds (or even longer) before you straighten your arms. This rhythm of muscle contraction is closer to what you experience in a fight, and it will allow you to use heavier weights.

Ⓑ The partial narrow-grip bench press, which consists of just the upper phase of the exercise (close to a complete extension of the arms), targets the triceps even more than a full bench press. This variation works on direct blows, such as hammer fists. In this case, the power of the strike primarily comes from the strength in the triceps.

These strikes are similar to a triceps extension, and doing partial narrow work will make you stronger in that exercise as well.

Ⓒ To train yourself to hit an opponent who is taller than you or to improve your uppercuts, use a slightly inclined bench.

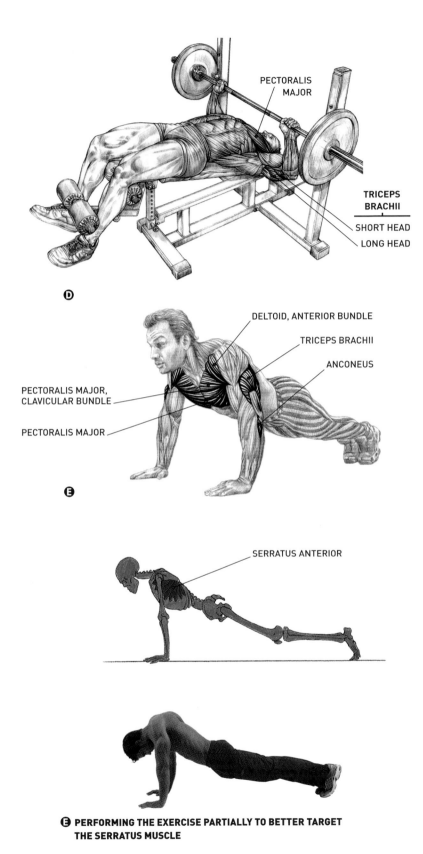

PECTORALIS MAJOR

**TRICEPS BRACHII**

SHORT HEAD

LONG HEAD

**Ⓓ**

DELTOID, ANTERIOR BUNDLE

TRICEPS BRACHII

ANCONEUS

PECTORALIS MAJOR, CLAVICULAR BUNDLE

PECTORALIS MAJOR

**Ⓔ**

SERRATUS ANTERIOR

**Ⓔ PERFORMING THE EXERCISE PARTIALLY TO BETTER TARGET THE SERRATUS MUSCLE**

**Ⓓ** To train yourself to hit an opponent who is shorter than you, or to hit him once he is on the ground, use a bench with a slight decline.

**Ⓔ** The narrow grip can be used in push-ups. Their major advantage over the bench press is that the shoulder blades are not immobilized on a bench. This forces the serratus anterior muscles to get involved in order to stabilize the shoulder blades. The serratus muscles also help project the arms forward, so these muscles can increase the power of your punches. To isolate the serratus anterior, or when you have reached fatigue doing push-ups, do a partial movement with straight arms by sinking down and making your shoulder blades stick out.

**Ⓕ** Instead of using a bench, put a padded cushion on the floor to get a slight elevation. This will let you push more with your thighs. Here, the goal is to mimic a defensive position when your back is on the floor. To make this exercise harder, squeeze a medicine ball between your legs during the set so that you also work your thighs. In fact, even on the floor, your arms work together with your legs.

## ADVANTAGES

This exercise is not specifically for fighters, but it is useful if you are just beginning strength training. It will help you quickly gain strength in your torso muscles.

## DISADVANTAGES

People rarely hit with both arms at the same time and especially not with the shoulder blades immobilized by a bench. Once you get stronger from doing narrow-grip bench presses, you should move on to an exercise that is specifically for fighting, which we describe next.

## ⚠ RISKS

The farther you extend, the more dangerous the bench press is for the chest and shoulder joints.

# PUNCH AND ELBOW STRIKE WITH ELASTIC BAND OR PULLEY

*This is a compound exercise for the triceps, chest, serratus anterior, shoulders, obliques, thighs, and calves.*

## WHY FIGHTERS SHOULD DO IT

★ To practice synchronizing muscle action and to increase the power of the four things that make punches stronger: support from the legs (calves, quadriceps, buttocks) plus torso rotation (obliques) plus thrusting the shoulder forward (serratus, deltoid, chest) plus extending the arms (triceps)

**Stand with a pulley or an elastic band behind you and grab the handle ❶. Get into a fighting stance and strike as violently as you can ❷ before returning to a defensive position. Do not keep doing repetitions mechanically; take a 1- to 2-second break in your defensive position between strikes. Once you have done a set on one arm, move to the other side without stopping to rest.**

## HELPFUL HINTS

Ideally, you should actually hit something, such as a BOSU ball ❸, rather than just punch the air.

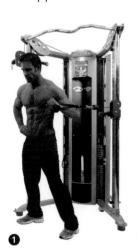

❶

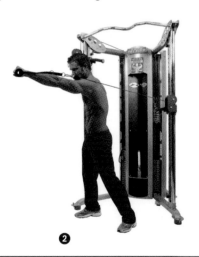

❷

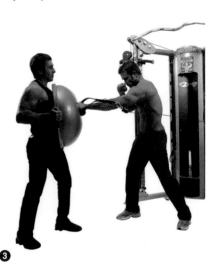

❸

## NOTES

Do this exercise with as much explosiveness as possible. The speed of the punch is more important than the resistance.

## VARIATIONS

**Ⓐ** Change your elbow position to work on different kinds of punches; do not practice just one kind.

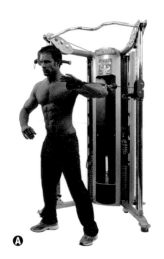

**Ⓐ**

**Ⓑ** If you use a low pulley, you can work on your uppercuts.

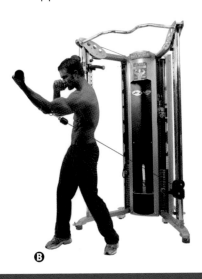

**Ⓑ**

**Ⓒ** If you put an elastic band around your back or use a double pulley, you can practice strikes with one arm and then the other or in a random fashion.

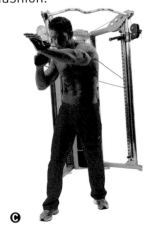

**Ⓒ**

**Ⓓ** Lean forward as if you were hitting an opponent on the floor.

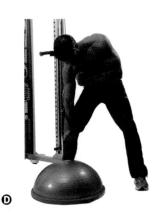

**Ⓓ**

**Ⓔ** Instead of standing up, kneel as if you were about to hit an opponent on the floor, ground-and-pound style.

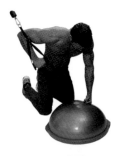

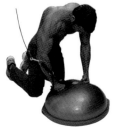

**Ⓔ Throwing a punch from a kneeling position**

**Ⓕ** Kneeling once again, practice elbow strikes as if you were hitting an opponent on the ground.

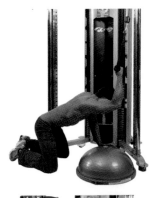

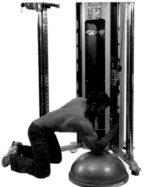

**Ⓕ Throwing an elbow strike from a kneeling position**

## ADVANTAGES

The direction of resistance is perfect. Compare this exercise to throwing punches with dumbbells in your hands, which works only the shoulders.

## DISADVANTAGES

There is no relaxation phase in this exercise. Of course, this means that you will also need to train using no resistance (with a punching bag).

## ⚠ RISKS

Since this really works the shoulder joint, make sure to warm it up well before any kind of punching work. A good warm-up is to do pulley shoulder rotations using an elastic band or a midlevel pulley.

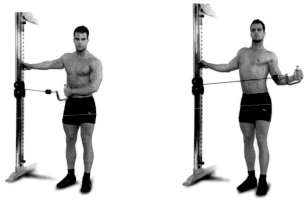

**PERFORMING SHOULDER ROTATIONS WITH A PULLEY**

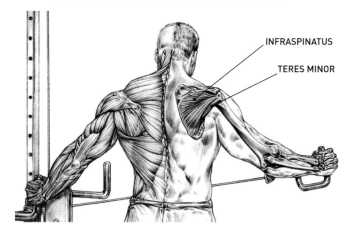

INFRASPINATUS

TERES MINOR

Doing pulley shoulder rotations is an excellent way to warm up the shoulder joint.

# MEDICINE BALL THROW

*This is a compound exercise for the triceps, shoulders, and abdominal wall.*

### WHY FIGHTERS SHOULD DO IT

★ To make your punches more explosive

You can combine sit-ups (see page 70) with a medicine ball throw. Hold the ball on your upper chest ❶, lift your torso, and throw the ball with as much power as you can ❷.

You must throw the ball before your torso reaches your knees.

A partner should stand near your feet to catch the ball and give it back to you before you begin to lower your torso.

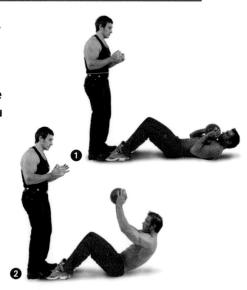

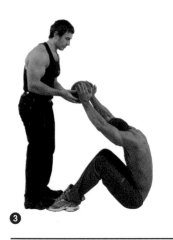

③

peculiarity when you do strength training.

## VARIATION
Instead of throwing the medicine ball straight ahead, rotate your torso and throw it to a partner who is standing at your left or right side. Ideally, your partner should switch sides each time so that you have to throw the ball in a different direction with every repetition.

## ADVANTAGES
This is a fun exercise that will improve the explosive power of your movements.

## DISADVANTAGES
Normally, you should train standing up, but then the exercise would not be as

effective for the abdominal wall.

## ⚠ RISKS
Never arch your back, even if it seems as though it gives you more stability when you throw.

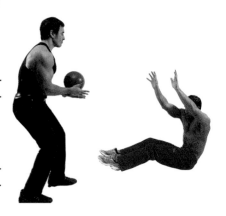

**ROTATING VARIATION**

## HELPFUL HINTS
Your partner needs to place the ball back in your hands ❸. Never have your partner throw the ball, because this kind of off-center repetition could damage your muscles and slow your muscle recovery. During a fight, there is almost no negative work when you throw a punch. You must respect this physiological

# FOREARMS

To prevent your fist from twisting upon impact, you need to strengthen your forearm extensor and flexor muscles to stabilize your wrist joint. Rigidity upon impact does not imply a lack of flexibility. It just means that at the moment your punch reaches your opponent, your forearm muscles are strong enough to prevent tiny movements in the wrist. These micromovements make a punch less effective and cause trauma to the joint. There are two exercises you can do for this: wrist extension and wrist curl.

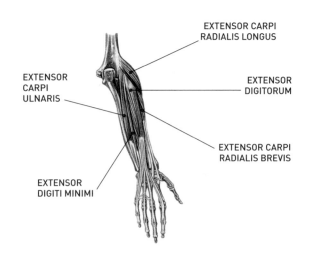

EXTENSOR CARPI RADIALIS LONGUS

EXTENSOR DIGITORUM

EXTENSOR CARPI RADIALIS BREVIS

EXTENSOR CARPI ULNARIS

EXTENSOR DIGITI MINIMI

*This is an isolation exercise for the outer part of the forearm.*

## WHY FIGHTERS SHOULD DO IT

★ To strengthen and stabilize the extensor muscles so that the wrist will not twist toward the inside at the moment of impact

Sit down and grab a bar (straight or twisted) or a dumbbell with your hands at either end. Use a pronated grip (thumbs facing each other) ❶. Rest your forearms on your thighs so that your hands hang free ❷. Use your forearms to lift your hands up ❸. Hold the contraction for 1 second before slowly lowering the weight.

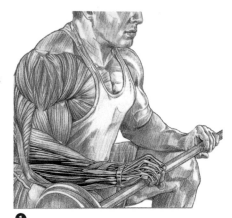

❶

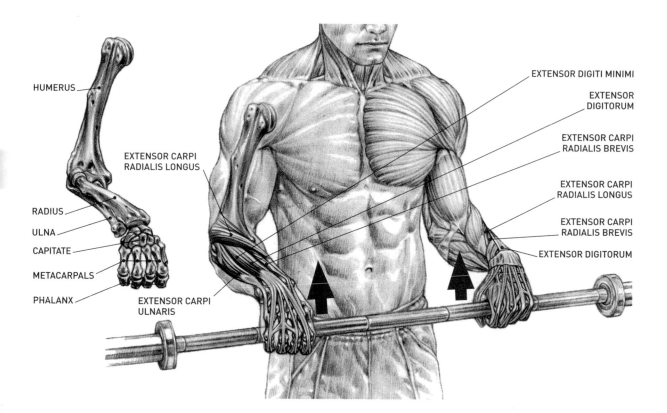

HUMERUS

EXTENSOR CARPI RADIALIS LONGUS

RADIUS

ULNA

CAPITATE

METACARPALS

PHALANX

EXTENSOR CARPI ULNARIS

EXTENSOR DIGITI MINIMI

EXTENSOR DIGITORUM

EXTENSOR CARPI RADIALIS BREVIS

EXTENSOR CARPI RADIALIS LONGUS

EXTENSOR CARPI RADIALIS BREVIS

EXTENSOR DIGITORUM

**MOTORCYCLE MOVEMENT DURING A WRIST EXTENSION**

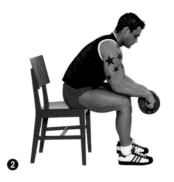

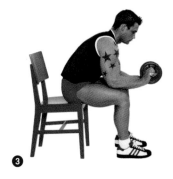

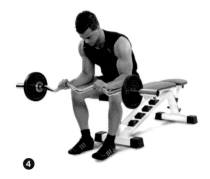

## HELPFUL HINTS

The straighter your arms are, the stronger you will be.

## ADVANTAGES

The extensor muscles are naturally weaker than the flexor muscles. Therefore, wrist extensions are the most important wrist

protection exercise that a fighter can do.

## DISADVANTAGES

Many people will have trouble holding a straight bar. Do not force your wrists by trying to imitate other people. A twisted bar ❹ will help you keep your thumbs a little higher than

your pinky fingers, which will prevent twisting in your wrist.

## ⚠ RISKS

Do not drop your wrists down too far at the bottom of the exercise, because this could overstretch your extensor muscles.

## WRIST CURL

**FLEXOR MUSCLES OF THE WRIST**

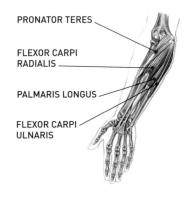

PRONATOR TERES

FLEXOR CARPI RADIALIS

PALMARIS LONGUS

FLEXOR CARPI ULNARIS

SUPERFICIAL LAYER

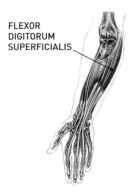

FLEXOR DIGITORUM SUPERFICIALIS

MIDDLE LAYER

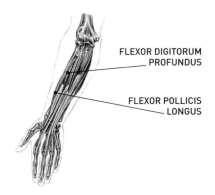

FLEXOR DIGITORUM PROFUNDUS

FLEXOR POLLICIS LONGUS

DEEP LAYER

*This is an isolation exercise for the inner part of the forearm.*

## WHY FIGHTERS SHOULD DO IT

★ To stabilize the wrists upon impact by strengthening the

flexor muscles. Strong and enduring flexor muscles will also help you effectively grab your opponents.

While seated, grab a bar (straight bar or EZ-bar) or a dumbbell at both ends in a supinated grip (thumbs toward the outside). Place your forearms on your thighs or on a bench so that your hands hang free ❶. Using your forearms, lift your hands as high as possible ❷. Hold the contraction for 1 second before slowly lowering the weight.

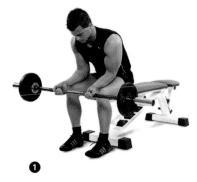

❶

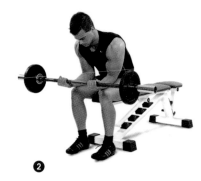

❷

## HELPFUL HINTS

The more you bend your arms, the stronger you will be during this exercise.

## VARIATIONS

❹ You can do wrist curls while standing up with a bar behind you using a pronated grip (thumbs facing each other). This variation is less dangerous for your wrists, so you can use a heavier weight.

❻ Keep the bar in front of your body or behind it, but instead of keeping your fist closed, open your hands up when your palms are perpendicular to the floor. Close your fists before doing another wrist curl. This variation strengthens your grip and works both the deep and superficial layers of the flexor muscles.

## ADVANTAGES

Wrist curls will help you dominate in grappling.

## DISADVANTAGES

The flexor muscles are naturally stronger than the extensor muscles. This means that wrist curls are less important than wrist extensions when it comes to protecting your forearms.

## ⚠ RISKS

Do not stretch too far in the lengthened position.

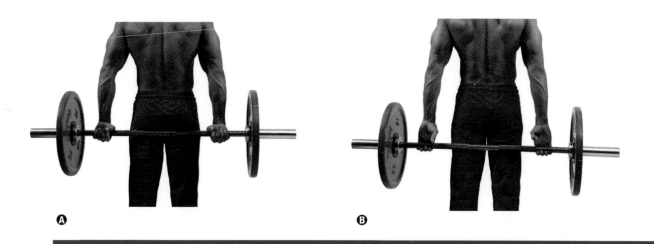

❹

❻

## PARTIAL SQUAT

*This is a compound exercise for the quadriceps, buttocks, hamstrings, lower back, and calves.*

### WHY FIGHTERS SHOULD DO IT

★ The thigh muscles play an important part in anchoring your body during a punch.

★ Squats will increase the power of your thrust during Superman punches or jumping knee kicks.

★ Doing heavy squats will help you push your opponent with more force during hand-to-hand fighting while standing up. You can use your strength to push your opponent backward.

★ By working the buttocks and hamstrings, squats improve your spinning kicks and stomp kicks.

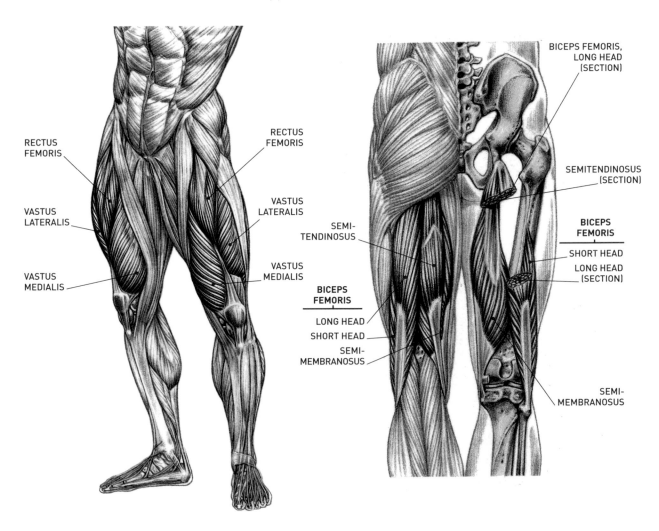

RECTUS FEMORIS

RECTUS FEMORIS

VASTUS LATERALIS

VASTUS LATERALIS

VASTUS MEDIALIS

VASTUS MEDIALIS

SEMI-TENDINOSUS

BICEPS FEMORIS

LONG HEAD

SHORT HEAD

SEMI-MEMBRANOSUS

BICEPS FEMORIS, LONG HEAD (SECTION)

SEMITENDINOSUS (SECTION)

BICEPS FEMORIS

SHORT HEAD

LONG HEAD (SECTION)

SEMI-MEMBRANOSUS

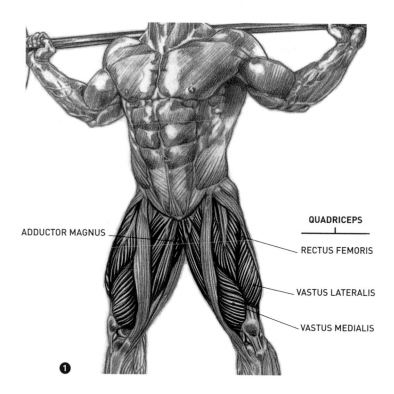

ADDUCTOR MAGNUS

QUADRICEPS

RECTUS FEMORIS

VASTUS LATERALIS

VASTUS MEDIALIS

**❶**

With your feet a bit narrower than shoulder-width apart, put a bar on the back of your shoulders (not on your neck). Keep your back flat and very slightly arched backward. Take one or two steps backward to get out of the rack. Keep your back as straight as possible and bend your legs. Go down 8 to 10 inches and then push through your legs until your legs are straight once again ❶.

## ⚠ WARNING!

Here is how you should hold your head: Look straight in front of you and slightly upward. If you look down, you could fall forward, which is very dangerous.

## HELPFUL HINTS

There is no point in trying to go down too low. The goal is to use as heavy a weight as possible over the usual range of motion that your thighs experience during a fight.

## ADVANTAGES

The squat works the entire lower body in a very short time.

## DISADVANTAGES

The longer your legs are, the more dangerous it is for your back to go down low. An awkward leg-to-torso ratio will make you bend very far forward, creating instability in your lower back (see page 27).

## ⚠ RISKS

In addition to warming up your knees, be sure to warm up your abdominal, oblique, and back muscles thoroughly to optimize your lumbar stability. As at the end of every workout that has compressed your spine, you should stretch out for a long time at the pull-up bar (see page 50).

## STANDING CALF RAISE

*This is an isolation exercise for the entire calf and lower back.*

### WHY FIGHTERS SHOULD DO IT

★ The strength in the calf muscles anchors the legs to the floor and allows you to strike effectively. The power of strikes thrown with the thigh or knee also depends on the calf being firmly anchored to the floor.

★ By getting stronger, your calf muscles will increase the power of your thrusts during Superman punches or jumping knee kicks.

★ When you are in a defensive clinch, powerful calf muscles will make the difference in your ability to push your opponent backward.

Select your weight and then get in the machine. Put the balls of your feet on the foot plate.

Stretch your calf muscles slightly before pushing up as high as you can onto the balls of your feet ❶. Hold the contracted position for 1 second before lowering to the lengthened position.

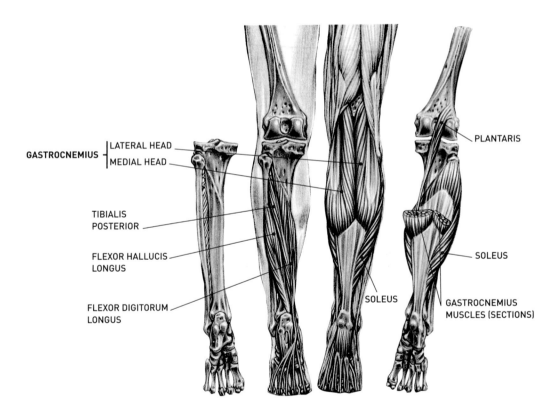

GASTROCNEMIUS — LATERAL HEAD
MEDIAL HEAD

TIBIALIS POSTERIOR

FLEXOR HALLUCIS LONGUS

FLEXOR DIGITORUM LONGUS

PLANTARIS

SOLEUS

SOLEUS

GASTROCNEMIUS MUSCLES (SECTIONS)

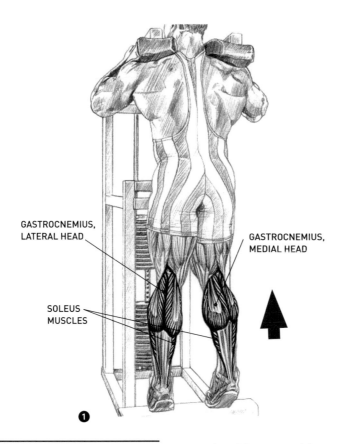

GASTROCNEMIUS, LATERAL HEAD

GASTROCNEMIUS, MEDIAL HEAD

SOLEUS MUSCLES

**①**

your legs to avoid any unnecessary twisting in your knees. The calves will also be strongest in this position. If you absolutely have to do a different version of the exercise, then you could change the width of your feet (close together or far apart) or work only one calf at a time.

## ADVANTAGES
This exercise works the entire calf.

## DISADVANTAGES
The calves rarely work together at the same time. You can work them individually, but that will take much more time.

## ⚠ RISKS
The heavier the weight you use, the more you compress your spine.

## HELPFUL HINTS
Avoid swinging your torso forward and backward while arching your lower back. This swinging is dangerous and is often caused by keeping your legs too straight, especially in the lengthened position.
   Keep your head straight and look very slightly upward.

## VARIATIONS
**Ⓐ** If you do not have the correct machine, you can do this exercise in a squat rack with the bar resting on

your shoulders or with dumbbells in your hands.

**Ⓑ** You can point your feet toward the outside or the inside, but it is better to keep them in line with

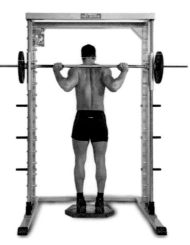

**Ⓐ USING A SQUAT RACK**

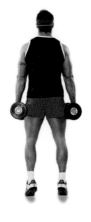

**Ⓐ USING DUMBBELLS**

# KICKS AND KNEE STRIKES

Surprising though it may seem, the power of kicks and knee strikes has very little to do with the thighs. The thighs actually slow down strikes. So if your thighs are really large, having to move their extra weight could also slow down your strikes. The power in kicks and knee strikes comes from the psoas and iliacus muscles. The rectus femoris is the only thigh muscle that supports the hip flexors. Stability, which keeps you from falling when you are standing on only one leg, is provided by the gluteus medius and calves. So these four groups of muscles are the ones you need to strengthen.

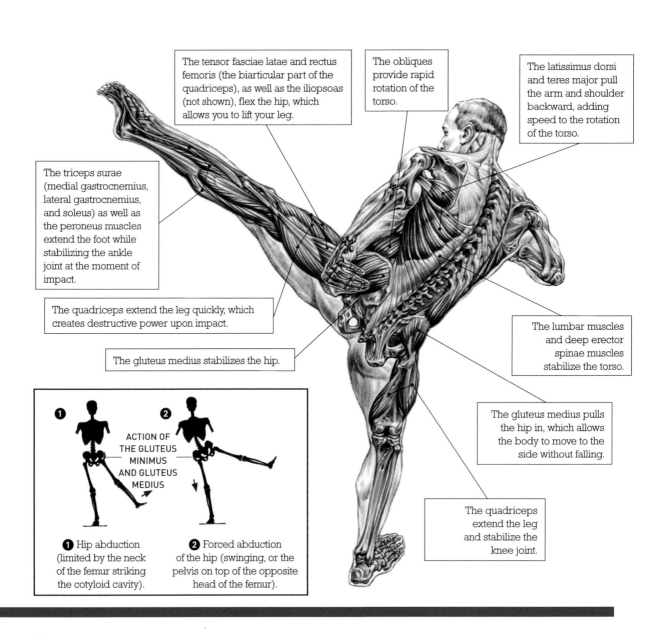

The tensor fasciae latae and rectus femoris (the biarticular part of the quadriceps), as well as the iliopsoas (not shown), flex the hip, which allows you to lift your leg.

The obliques provide rapid rotation of the torso.

The latissimus dorsi and teres major pull the arm and shoulder backward, adding speed to the rotation of the torso.

The triceps surae (medial gastrocnemius, lateral gastrocnemius, and soleus) as well as the peroneus muscles extend the foot while stabilizing the ankle joint at the moment of impact.

The quadriceps extend the leg quickly, which creates destructive power upon impact.

The gluteus medius stabilizes the hip.

The lumbar muscles and deep erector spinae muscles stabilize the torso.

The gluteus medius pulls the hip in, which allows the body to move to the side without falling.

The quadriceps extend the leg and stabilize the knee joint.

ACTION OF THE GLUTEUS MINIMUS AND GLUTEUS MEDIUS

❶ Hip abduction (limited by the neck of the femur striking the cotyloid cavity).

❷ Forced abduction of the hip (swinging, or the pelvis on top of the opposite head of the femur).

Scientific research shows that about 60% of the psoas major is composed of fast-twitch (type 2) fibers. Yet in humans, the type 1 fibers are larger. This paradox highlights the fact that we are not using common sense to work this muscle because, normally, type 2 fibers are always larger than type 1 fibers. So if the slow-twitch fibers in the psoas are hypertrophied, it means that only the postural support function of the muscle is being used. This means that a lack of stimulation is obtained through heavy, explosive exercises. A fighter who strikes with the legs must absolutely correct this deficiency.

To be able to strike with your legs as aggressively as possible, you must work your hip flexors using very heavy weights. Their physiological function requires this because of the vast number of fast-twitch fibers they contain.

## ⚠ WARNING!

Even though it is essential for you as a fighter to work the psoas and iliacus muscles intensively, this does not come without its own set of problems. This is the second paradox of the hip flexors. Working them can have two negative consequences:

1. In the short term, some exercises can hurt your discs.
2. In the long term, overtoned flexors can create an arch in the lower spine. This poor spinal position, coupled with the intense pressure that strength training places on the vertebrae, can dramatically increase your risk of a lower back injury.

To prevent these problems, you must do the following:

→ Stretch the psoas and iliacus by doing lunges after you have worked them ❶.
→ Hang from a pull-up bar to decompress your lumbar spine (see page 50).

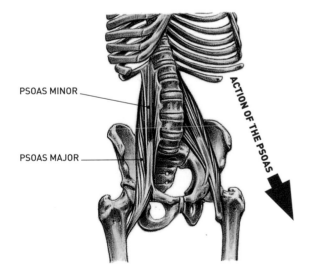

PSOAS MINOR

PSOAS MAJOR

ACTION OF THE PSOAS

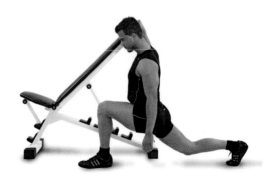

❶ STRETCHING THE PSOAS AND ILIACUS

## STANDING LEG LIFT

*This is an isolation exercise for the rectus femoris, psoas, iliacus, and abdominal muscles as well as the gluteus medius and calves.*

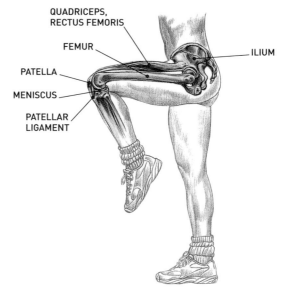

QUADRICEPS, RECTUS FEMORIS

FEMUR

ILIUM

PATELLA

MENISCUS

PATELLAR LIGAMENT

### WHY FIGHTERS SHOULD DO IT

★ To focus specifically on the muscles that make your kicks and knee strikes more powerful. It will also improve your balance, which is always problematic when standing on one leg.

**Stand up and put a weight plate or a dumbbell on your left thigh a little above the knee ❶. Stabilize the weight with your left hand and use your right hand to hold on to a machine or wall to ensure your balance. Lift your leg as high as you can while bending your knee ❷. Then lower your leg until your thigh is perpendicular to the floor. Once you have done a set on the left leg, move on to the right leg.**

### HELPFUL HINTS

You can rest your foot on the floor between repetitions. This midset break will allow you to use heavier weights.

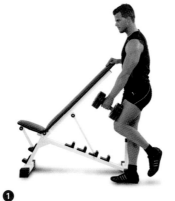

❶

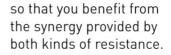

❷

### VARIATIONS

❹ Instead of using a dumbbell, you can wrap an elastic band around your leg just above your knee. Put the other end under the foot that is resting on the floor.

❺ You can also combine an elastic band and a weight so that you benefit from the synergy provided by both kinds of resistance.

❻ To work on the stabilization muscles (gluteus medius and calf), use your free hand for balance less and less (or perhaps not at all).

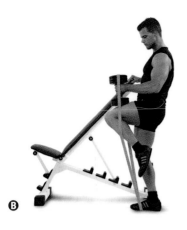

**B**

**D** Instead of bending your leg as you lift it, keep it straight throughout the exercise.

**E** There are machines specifically designed for leg lifts. Though they are easier to use than dumbbells since you are perfectly balanced, they are not very helpful for fighters.

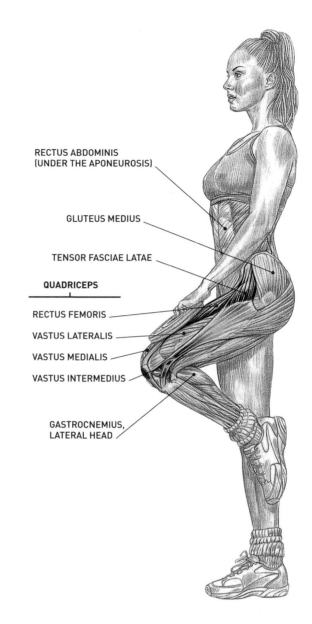

RECTUS ABDOMINIS
(UNDER THE APONEUROSIS)

GLUTEUS MEDIUS

TENSOR FASCIAE LATAE

**QUADRICEPS**

RECTUS FEMORIS

VASTUS LATERALIS

VASTUS MEDIALIS

VASTUS INTERMEDIUS

GASTROCNEMIUS,
LATERAL HEAD

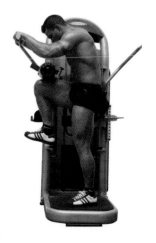

**E**

### ADVANTAGES
Leg lifts work muscles that are often neglected even though they are essential in a fight.

### DISADVANTAGES
Since this exercise must be done unilaterally, it will take you more time to complete.

### ⚠ RISKS
Working the psoas pulls on the spine. Keep your back very straight and be careful not to arch your lower back. If you feel any movement in your spine, do not lift your thigh up as high.

*This is an isolation exercise for the rectus femoris, psoas, iliacus, abdominal muscles, and arms.*

### WHY FIGHTERS SHOULD DO IT

★ To train yourself to perform knee strikes and kicks with your arms contracted, as when you grab your opponent's neck with your hands so you can strike better.

**Grab a pull-up bar using a supinated grip (pinky fingers facing each other) with your hands about shoulder-width apart. Pull with your biceps so that you bend your arms ❶ and bend your right leg to bring your knee toward your chin ❷. Lift your leg as high as you can as you tilt your pelvis up. Then lower your leg.**

**Once you have done a repetition on the right leg, switch to the left leg. If your arms get tired before your legs, rest your feet on the floor and end the set using a pronated grip (thumbs facing each other).**

### HELPFUL HINTS

When you first do this exercise, the hardest part will be trying not to swing back and forth because

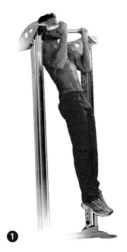

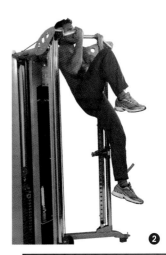

only your arms provide stability. As you continue training, you will learn to hold your body still.

### VARIATIONS

❹ You can do one of the following:
– Keep your legs straight (the exercise will be much harder this way).
– Bring your calves under your thighs (this will make the exercise easier).

❺ When the exercise becomes too easy, you can add resistance by using an ankle weight or an elastic band attached to the floor and wrapped around your leg just above your knee. But when using an elastic band, you will not be able to alternate legs as you do the exercise.

### ADVANTAGES

The resistance placed on all these muscles is at the maximum, which means you will progress quickly.

### DISADVANTAGES

A pulling sensation in your lower back means you are doing the exercise incorrectly. A learning period is probably required.

### ⚠ RISKS

Do not arch your lower back.

*This is an isolation exercise for the rectus femoris, psoas, iliacus, and abdominal muscles.*

## WHY FIGHTERS SHOULD DO IT

★ To get stronger when doing knee strikes on the ground when you have side control.

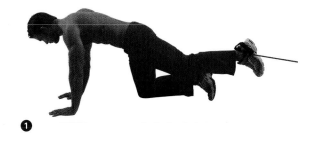

**Attach an elastic band or the cable of a low pulley around your left ankle. Get on all fours ❶. Bring your left knee forward as if you were doing a knee strike on an opponent lying down ❷.**

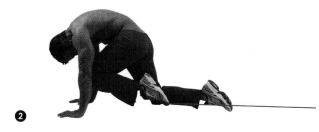

### HELPFUL HINTS

Ideally, you should hold a BOSU ball with your hands and strike it so you can train your muscle to increase its contraction at the moment of impact.

### VARIATION

When you are doing knee strikes on the ground, it is common to use your arms to choke your opponent. To reproduce this fighting position better, grab a machine or the BOSU ball with your hands as firmly as you can.

### ADVANTAGES

This exercise accurately reproduces the position used in a fight.

### DISADVANTAGES

Once you have finished working one leg, you have to reposition the elastic band on the other leg, which may become tedious.

### ⚠ RISKS

Do not arch backward. On the contrary, you should round your back to prevent disc problems.

# GRABS, PULLS, AND CHOKES

When you have to pull, knock off balance, or choke an opponent, your arms are the most important. They are seconded by your back. To be able to grab an opponent and hold on, you need to strengthen your forearms and hands.

## PULL-UP

*This is a compound exercise for the forearm flexors and back muscles. The accent is placed on both the contraction and the static portions of the exercise.*

### WHY FIGHTERS SHOULD DO IT

★ To strengthen the arms and back muscles, which are indispensable when you are pulling an opponent toward you in order to knock the competitor off balance
★ To increase the power of your guillotine choke

**Grab the pull-up bar with a supinated grip (pinky fingers facing each other) ❶. Your hands should be a bit narrower than shoulder-width apart. Lift yourself using the strength in your back and arms ❷. The top of the exercise is when your chin reaches the bar. Hold that contracted position for 5 seconds before coming back down.**

### VARIATIONS

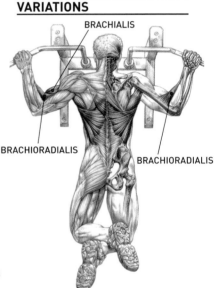

**Ⓐ PRONATED GRIP**

Ⓐ To alternate the muscle work in your arms, you can use a pronated grip (thumbs facing each other), which stimulates the brachioradialis, or a neutral grip (thumbs facing your torso), which stimulates the brachialis.

Ⓑ Once pull-ups become too easy, add some resistance with a weight.

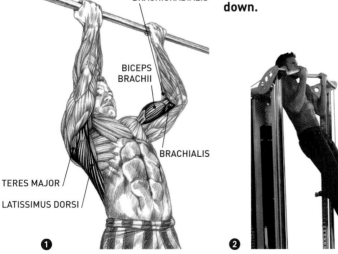

BRACHIORADIALIS

BICEPS BRACHII

BRACHIALIS

TERES MAJOR

LATISSIMUS DORSI

❶

❷

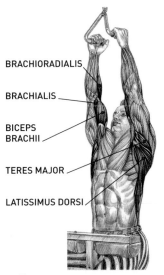

BRACHIORADIALIS

BRACHIALIS

BICEPS
BRACHII

TERES MAJOR

LATISSIMUS DORSI

**Ⓐ NEUTRAL GRIP (HIGH PULLEY WITH A HANDLE USING A CLOSE GRIP)**

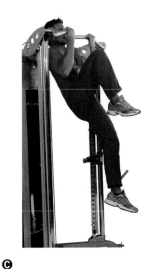

**Ⓒ**

**Ⓒ** When you pull an opponent toward you, you often take the opportunity to do some knee strikes. Instead of keeping your legs still during this exercise, take this time to

train yourself to do knee strikes while your arms are working.

## ADVANTAGES

Pull-ups work numerous muscles in the torso in a short time and require very little equipment.

## DISADVANTAGES

Unfortunately, not everyone can do pull-ups. If you are not strong enough, rest your feet on the floor or on a chair to make the exercise easier.

## ⚠ RISKS

Do not straighten your arms completely when your hands are supinated (pinky fingers facing each other), or you could injure your biceps.

# POWER TRICEPS PUSH-DOWN

*This is a compound exercise that focuses on the triceps and back.*

## WHY FIGHTERS SHOULD DO IT

★ To get stronger so you can knock an opponent off balance by pulling him toward you so that he falls forward or so that you can choke him against your torso

**Attach a cord or triceps bar to a high pulley. Face the machine and use your**

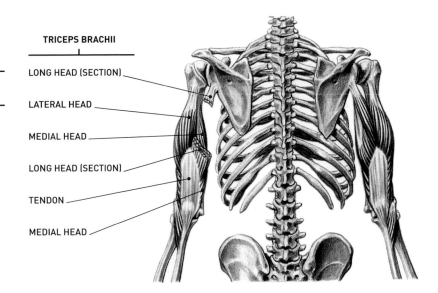

TRICEPS BRACHII

LONG HEAD (SECTION)

LATERAL HEAD

MEDIAL HEAD

LONG HEAD (SECTION)

TENDON

MEDIAL HEAD

triceps to push down **❶ ❷**. Instead of keeping your upper arms and elbows at your sides as in the standard version, lift them in parallel position with the hands. Instead of stopping at the lower chest, the cord comes up toward the neck so that your upper arms are almost parallel to the floor at the end of the lengthened phase of the exercise. To do the exercise explosively, use your back and triceps muscles to bring the bar or cord to your upper thighs.

> **★ TIP:** Use your body weight in addition to your muscles as if you were trying to bury an opponent in the ground.

### HELPFUL HINTS
Because of the explosive aspect of this exercise, use an adjustable pulley if you can. The weights on a triceps machine could be too light.

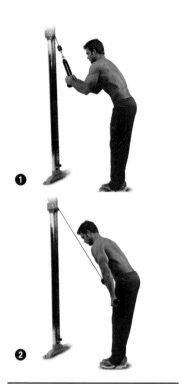

**❶**

**❷**

### VARIATION
You can do this exercise on your knees to prepare yourself for wrestling on the ground.

### NOTES
The bigger the bar or cord that you use, the stronger you will feel and the easier this exercise will be on your elbows. Bars that are

1 inch (2.5 cm) in diameter are common, but these are too small to train you to grab an opponent's arm effectively. To increase the diameter of these bars, you can hold sponges between your hands and the bar.

### ADVANTAGES
Using a cable pulley is easier on your elbows than doing the exercise with dumbbells, a bar, or machines.

### DISADVANTAGES
When using heavy weights, it is hard to keep your feet firmly on the floor. If this happens to you, slip one foot under a very heavy dumbbell.

### ⚠ RISKS
Do not arch your back. Also, be careful not to scratch your face because the cable is passing right by your head.

## HANG FROM PULL-UP BAR

*This is an isolation exercise for the wrist flexors, especially the deep flexor muscles of the forearms.*

### WHY FIGHTERS SHOULD DO IT
★ To improve gripping strength in every situation. In free

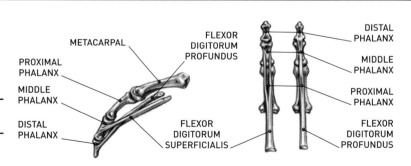

**INSERTION OF THE FINGER FLEXOR MUSCLES ON THE PHALANGES**

fighting, having strong forearms is even more important than in judo, because when there is no uniform stance, you have to grab your opponent's arm. Because of the size of that arm, the rounded shape, and the sweat, it is not easy to maintain a good grip.

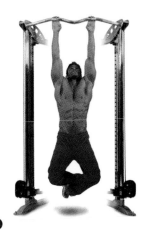

**Hang from a pull-up bar with straight arms and a pronated grip (thumbs facing each other) ❶. You can place your hands where it feels the most comfortable for you. Open your hands slightly, but do not let go of the bar ❷. After lowering down about 2 inches (5 cm), come back up by using your fingers to close your grip around the bar. Hold the contraction for 5 to 10 seconds before opening your hands again slowly.**

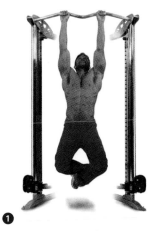

## HELPFUL HINTS
Even when you no longer have enough strength to open your hands, you will certainly have enough to hold yourself suspended from the bar with a closed grip for 10 seconds or so.

## NOTES
High-level fighters have just 8% greater hand strength than people who do strength training but do not especially focus on their wrists. They

are far behind baseball players, who have greater hand strength than MMA champions. So fighters have a lot of catching up to do in their forearms. Doing this exercise at the pull-up bar is an excellent way to overcome this strength deficit.

## VARIATIONS
❹ If you have trouble opening your hands, lighten your body weight by resting one or even both feet on the floor or on a chair.

❸ When the exercise becomes too easy, do it unilaterally by hanging from only one hand. The other arm will be used only to stabilize your body side to side.

## ADVANTAGES
This is an easy exercise that strengthens the hand grip.

## DISADVANTAGES
Be careful not to create problems in your hands by opening your fingers too abruptly.

## ⚠ RISKS
As you approach failure, keep your feet close to the floor to avoid a sudden fall in case you accidentally let go of the bar.

*This isolation exercise works all the forearm flexors: biceps, brachialis, and brachioradialis. The focus should be on the contraction as well as the static phase of the exercise.*

## WHY FIGHTERS SHOULD DO IT

★ To gain isometric muscular endurance in the forearm flexors to make your chokes and arm locks more effective

**Grab a dumbbell with your hand in the neutral position (thumb pointing up). Bend your arm and keep your thumb pointing up ❶. Lift the dumbbell as high as possible. To do this, you can pull your elbow back slightly, but be careful not to move it too much. Hold the contraction for 5 seconds. Slowly lower to the starting position.**

## VARIATIONS

**❹** You can do this exercise while standing or sitting (to work as if you were fighting on the ground).

**❺** There are several ways to do this exercise:

– With both hands at the same time
– By lifting one arm and then the other to

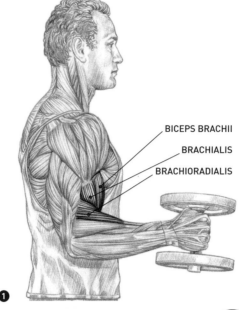

BICEPS BRACHII
BRACHIALIS
BRACHIORADIALIS

❶

alternate repetitions
– Using only one arm for an entire set

**❻** From one set to the next, change the position of your thumb so that you work your flexors from different angles:

– When your thumbs face the outside, the biceps will intervene more in the exercise.
– When your thumbs face the inside, the brachioradialis will work more and the biceps will work less.

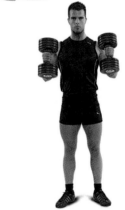

**❺ WITH BOTH ARMS TOGETHER**

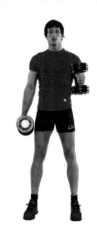

**❺ ALTERNATING ARMS**

# CHOKES AND COUNTERMOVES

When you choke an opponent, you use every muscle in your body. However, your arms play the biggest part. In your legs, your adductors and shins do most of the work.

Chokes and countermoves differ from other movements because even though the contraction is intense, the movement itself is slow, almost static. This is why it is so important to train with isometrics.

## EXERCISES FOR ENDURANCE

### HANG FROM STRAPS

*This is an isolation exercise for the biceps, forearms, back, and chest. It is done isometrically.*

**WHY FIGHTERS SHOULD DO IT**

★ To gain static muscular endurance in your arms so that you can crush your opponent during a choke

**Stand up and place your forearms in two ab straps ❶. Once your arms are ready, bend your legs so that you are hanging by your arms ❷. At first, do not hold on to your forearms with your hands. As you get tired, you can use your hands so that you can continue the exercise. Hold the position for at least 30 seconds. Then rest for 10 to 15 seconds before doing another repetition.**

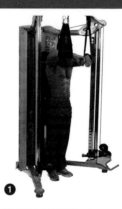
❶

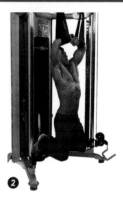
❷

★ **TIP:** When you can easily hang for more than 30 seconds, add some weights to your body or ask a partner to pull on your legs to make the exercise harder.

**HELPFUL HINTS**

If you do not have ab straps, you can make a loop with a judo belt. Use two belts on each arm because a single belt is too narrow and will hurt your arms.

**VARIATIONS**

Ⓐ During a choke with your arms, you often do knee strikes on your opponent. Rather than keep your legs

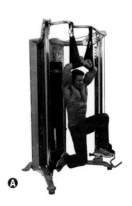
Ⓐ

bent, you can practice doing knee strikes while you are suspended.

**B** Instead of hanging from your forearms, you can place the straps around your upper arms to recruit your back muscles more.

**C** If you squeeze a large medicine ball between your thighs, you can prepare yourself to choke simultaneously with your arms and thighs.

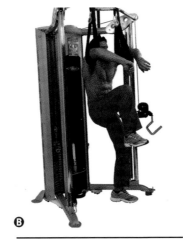

**B**

### ADVANTAGES

This is a static exercise that accurately reproduces the

contraction required for a choke with the arms.

### DISADVANTAGES

The strength orientation is not exactly the same as it would be in an actual fight, but this exercise will still provide gripping strength that will help you during a choke.

## ISOMETRIC ADDUCTION

*This is an isolation exercise that works the adductors isometrically, just as in a fight.*

### WHY FIGHTERS SHOULD DO IT

★ To gain static muscular endurance in the adductors so that you can crush your opponent with your thighs during a choke on the ground. The adductors are also involved when you do side kicks to buckle your opponent's leg.

**Lie on the floor holding a medicine ball (the biggest one you can find) between your legs ❶. Place it just above your knees, toward your thigh.**

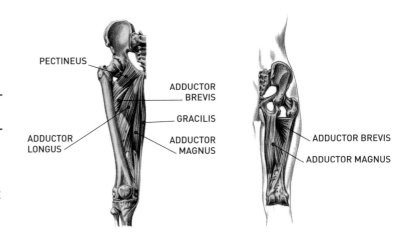

PECTINEUS

ADDUCTOR BREVIS

GRACILIS

ADDUCTOR LONGUS

ADDUCTOR MAGNUS

ADDUCTOR BREVIS

ADDUCTOR MAGNUS

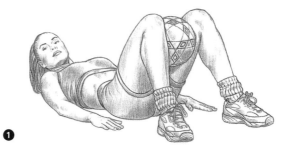

**❶**

**Squeeze as hard as you can, as if you were trying to pop the ball. Hold for at least 30 seconds. Rest for 10 to 15 seconds between repetitions.**

> ★ **TIP:** If you do not have a medicine ball, you can use a basketball.

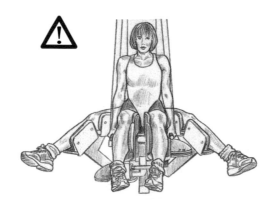

Be careful when using adductor machines. Some of them can increase the risk of knee injuries.

### HELPFUL HINTS

The angles you are working isometrically should be as close as possible to the ones used when squeezing an opponent during a fight.

### NOTES

High-level fighters have 44% greater strength in their adductors than people who do only strength training (Keating et al., 2011, *Journal of Strength and Conditioning Research,* 25:S50-1). This strength does not happen naturally; you must work to develop it.

### VARIATIONS

**Ⓐ** Once you can easily squeeze the ball for longer than 30 seconds, you can ask a partner to push the medicine ball toward the floor so that you will have to squeeze your legs together even harder.

**Ⓑ** During a choke, the level of thigh flexion varies. You need to replicate this diversity by bending your legs to varying degrees, so you can do this exercise with your legs almost straight or bent to 45 or 90 degrees.

**Ⓒ** Instead of lying on the floor, you can do this exercise on all fours.

### ADVANTAGES

This is a static exercise that accurately replicates the orientation of strength during a choke on the ground.

### DISADVANTAGES

A medicine ball cannot struggle the way an opponent can. But if your adductors are strong enough, you can paralyze your opponent by squeezing your muscles.

### ⚠ RISKS

There are adductor exercises and machines that place resistance on the ankle or the foot. This is generally the case for people who do the exercise with straight legs. This way they work the adductor magnus and the gracilis in proper alignment, which reproduces the muscle contraction that occurs in a high kick.

But by doing this, they could also tear the ligaments in the knee that facilitate the movement of the meniscus toward the inside. Placing the resistance low increases the risk of pinching the meniscus between the two condyles, which is both painful and debilitating.

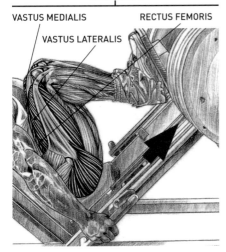

QUADRICEPS

VASTUS MEDIALIS

RECTUS FEMORIS

VASTUS LATERALIS

*This is a compound exercise for the quadriceps, buttocks, hamstrings, and calves.*

## WHY FIGHTERS SHOULD DO IT

★ If your back is on the floor and your opponent is standing at your feet trying to land on top of you to hit you, you can use your legs to kick off your opponent. The leg press using full range of motion will give you the strength required to do this effectively.

★ Unlike the slow movements done in the other exercises in this section, here you need to work explosively. The leg press will also improve your stomp kicks.

Select your weight and then get in the machine. Place your feet on the foot plate about shoulder-width apart ❶. Push with your thighs and disengage the safeties. Keep your back straight and pressed into the cushion. Lower the foot plate, using your thighs to slow the movement ❷. Lower the plate until you feel your lower back start to come up off the cushion.

Then push with your legs until they are almost straight. Repeat until fatigued.

## HELPFUL HINTS

When doing the leg press, the lower down you go, the more your back tends to come off the cushion. Once your back is off the cushion, your strength and range of motion in the exercise will improve. However, this comes at the price of increasing your risk of a lower back injury. This is why you should not arch your back.

## ADVANTAGES

The leg press recruits the entire lower body in a short time and in a position that is similar to what you experience in a fight. Compared to squats,

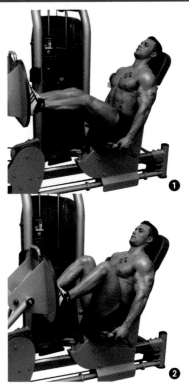

with the leg press your back is better protected in the machine. The machine also provides stability, which is an important safety measure.

## DISADVANTAGES

This exercise can be dangerous for the back, hips, and knees.

## ⚠ RISKS

Even if the spine appears to be held in place by the cushion of the machine, it is still subjected to enormous pressure.

## SEATED SQUAT

*This is a compound exercise for the entire thigh.*

### WHY FIGHTERS SHOULD DO IT

★ To be able to get up when you are sitting with your back against the cage and an opponent is trying to choke you

**Sit with your back against a wall and hold a dumbbell in your hands in the crease of your thighs. Stand up as quickly as you can.**

### HELPFUL HINTS

Get used to doing this exercise with no weight.

Then you can add weight until you get strong enough so that you can stand up during a fight no matter what happens.

### VARIATION

Without weight, you can stand up using just one leg instead of both. In this case, your other leg will help you to balance. Do a repetition on one leg and then switch to the other one.

### ADVANTAGES

This is an excellent exercise, but it's only for cage fighters.

### DISADVANTAGES

Unlike a dumbbell, an opponent can react and try to prevent you from standing back up. But if you have become strong enough from doing this exercise, your opponent will only be able to slow you down; he will not be able to stop you.

### ⚠ RISKS

Be careful of your knees. Because you start from an extremely low position, the knees are worked very hard.

## LYING LEG CURL

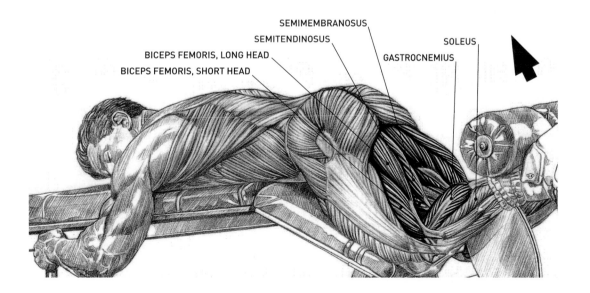

SEMIMEMBRANOSUS
SEMITENDINOSUS
BICEPS FEMORIS, LONG HEAD
BICEPS FEMORIS, SHORT HEAD
GASTROCNEMIUS
SOLEUS

*This is an isolation exercise for the hamstrings. It is best to do this exercise unilaterally, because in the holds described, only one leg is used at a time.*

## WHY FIGHTERS SHOULD DO IT

★ To choke your opponent's head between your calf and the back of your leg, you need strong static muscular endurance in your hamstring.

★ When you are standing and you hook your opponent's leg with your foot to make him fall, you need a powerful hamstring to accomplish the maneuver.

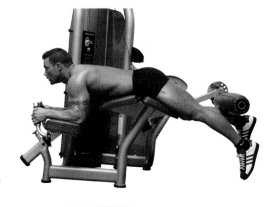

❶

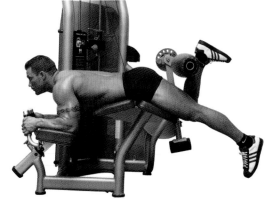

❷

**Select your weight and lie facedown on the machine. Put one ankle under the padded cushion ❶.**

**Use your hamstring to bring your foot up toward your buttocks ❷. Hold the contracted position for 5 to 10 seconds before lowering to the lengthened position.**

**Switch feet and do a repetition with the other leg. Continue alternating repetitions until you get tired.**

## HELPFUL HINTS

If the padded cushion rolls too much on your ankles or if it slides off when you are in the lengthened position, this means that the leg lever is not adjusted correctly.

## NOTES

The placement of the toes is important for a fighter. By flexing the toes toward your knees, you will be stronger since your calves will work together with your thighs. In addition, you will work the shin, a very important muscle for fighting, as you will see next.

## VARIATION

When working unilaterally, use the hand closest to the machine to push on the weights and make the exercise harder during the isometric contraction.

## ADVANTAGES

Since this exercise isolates the hamstring, it is relatively easy to do.

## ⚠ RISKS

If you arch your back, you will be stronger, but you will also compress your lower back.

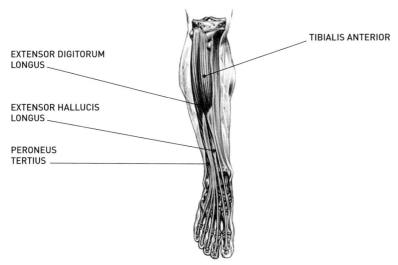

EXTENSOR DIGITORUM LONGUS

EXTENSOR HALLUCIS LONGUS

PERONEUS TERTIUS

TIBIALIS ANTERIOR

*This isolation exercise works the tibialis anterior isometrically, just as in a fight.*

### WHY FIGHTERS SHOULD DO IT

★ On the ground, to choke an opponent, make a triangle with your legs. Often, you use the top of your foot as an anchor point by pinning it against your calf or your opponent's thigh. Your opponent will then be perfectly immobilized, provided that the muscle on your shin has enough static muscular endurance.

★ The tibialis anterior also protects the tibia and makes any strike with the calf or the top of the foot more powerful.

**Find a stationary point, such as a weight machine, under which you can tuck your feet. Place your feet so they point slightly toward each other. Support yourself on your heels and the top part of your toes. Lean backward and hold this isometric contraction for at least 30 seconds. Rest for 10 to 15 seconds between repetitions.**

### HELPFUL HINTS

At first, use your hands for stability. Once you have become stronger, try not to use your hands. Put a folded towel between your feet and the support to prevent discomfort. However, be careful that your feet do not slide out of the machine.

### VARIATIONS

**A** As soon as you gain some endurance, stop using both feet and try the exercise with only one foot at a time.

**B** During a choke, the level of flexion in the thigh varies quite a bit. You should try to replicate this variability by bending your leg more or less, so you can do the exercise standing up with almost-straight legs, with legs bent to 45 or 90 degrees, or while seated on the floor.

### ADVANTAGES

Despite its importance in ground chokes, the tibialis anterior muscle is often neglected.

### DISADVANTAGES

You must have a solid anchor point to be able to do this exercise.

### ⚠ RISKS

Be careful that your foot does not slip out, or you will fall.

*This is an isolation exercise for the buttocks, lower back, and hamstrings.*

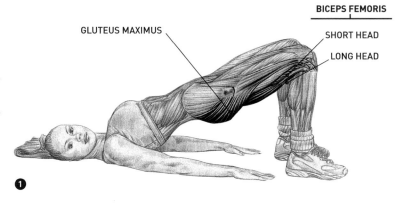

GLUTEUS MAXIMUS

BICEPS FEMORIS

SHORT HEAD

LONG HEAD

❶

## WHY FIGHTERS SHOULD DO IT

★ When you are on your back and an opponent has you in a choke hold on the floor, you have to be able to push up on your buttocks if you want to throw your opponent off of you. This way you can get out of the hold and maybe even reverse the situation.

**Lie down with your arms alongside your body and your feet about shoulder-width apart. Bend your legs to 90 degrees to bring your heels toward your buttocks.**

**Use your buttocks to lift your torso and legs up as high as you can to make a triangle with the floor. Your shoulders should stay in contact with the floor and serve as a lever ❶.**

**Hold the contracted position for 1 second and squeeze your buttocks as hard as you can. Return to the starting position and then do another repetition.**

## ⚠ WARNING!

Unlike the woman in the illustration, you should not turn your head to the side. Instead, look at the ceiling to protect your cervical spine.

## HELPFUL HINTS

To get better at pushing someone off of you and to have the advantage of surprise, you need to lift your pelvis up as quickly and explosively as you can.

## VARIATIONS

❶ Place your feet closer or farther away from your butt and vary the width of your feet. This will replicate the various situations you will encounter in a fight.

❷ Make this exercise more difficult by holding a large weight or by having

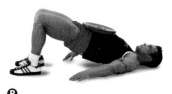

❸

your partner sit on your abdomen. You could even have your partner sit on your abdomen while holding a weight.

## ADVANTAGES

This position is very similar to what you experience in a fight.

## DISADVANTAGES

This exercise is easy to do, and that is why you need to train with as heavy a weight as you can handle.

## ⚠ RISKS

Do not arch your back just so you can raise your torso higher, because this could pinch the discs in your lumbar and cervical spine.

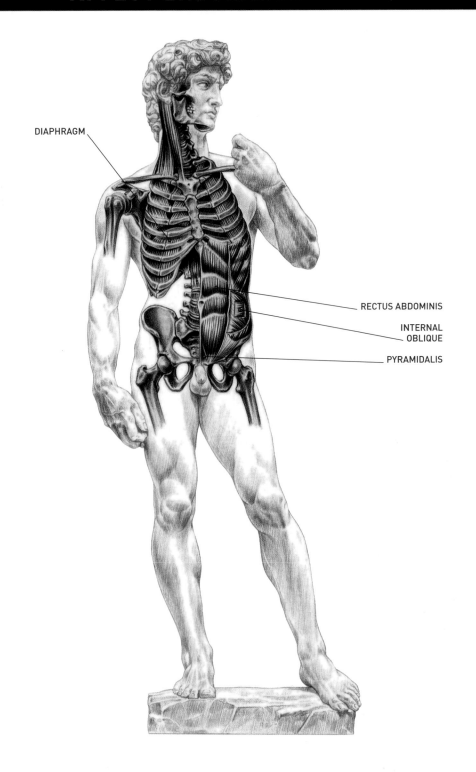

DIAPHRAGM

RECTUS ABDOMINIS

INTERNAL
OBLIQUE

PYRAMIDALIS

Scientific research has shown that during an endurance activity, the muscles used for breathing, especially the diaphragm, become fatigued. Just as with other muscles, this fatigue causes decreased performance. However, strength training exercises for the diaphragm can profoundly improve endurance.

For example, runners who warm up their breathing muscles before a race can increase their endurance by 5% to 7%. Spending 4 weeks training those breathing muscles can increase endurance by 12% (Lomax et al., 2011, *Journal of Sports Sciences*, 29(6):563-9). High-level athletes typically have larger diaphragms than their sedentary counterparts. So fighters should train their breathing muscles to prevent shortness of breath.

## LYING RIB CAGE EXPANSION WITH WEIGHT

*By making the expansion of the rib cage more difficult, this isolation exercise strengthens all the muscles that control inhalation.*

### WHY FIGHTERS SHOULD DO IT

★ To keep from getting tired during a fight and to get used to breathing even when your rib cage is compressed by the body weight of an opponent who is pinning you on the ground

**Lie on your back and put a dumbbell ❶ or a weight plate ❷ on your chest. Inhale deeply so that you expand your rib cage to its maximum, and then exhale to contract your rib cage.**

### HELPFUL HINTS

This exercise will do nothing for your endurance unless you do it in long sets (at least 50 repetitions).

### NOTES

Put a folded towel between the weight and your chest to prevent discomfort. This way you can train with the heaviest weight possible.

### VARIATIONS

❶ A partner can sit on your rib cage to provide resistance. Just be sure he sits down as gently as possible and not abruptly.

❷ Wear a mouth guard when you do this exercise, which will affect your breathing even more.

### ⚠ RISKS

Do not start with a heavy weight that will crush your ribs. Start with a light weight so your rib cage can get used to this exercise.

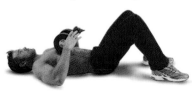

❶

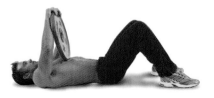

❷

When your back is on the ground during a fight, you need flexibility in your hip rotators and buttocks so that you can perform these moves:

→ Slide one leg up as high as possible to perform an omoplata.

→ Grab your opponent's head for a triangle or other choke.

Strength training exercises make the hips more rigid, but the hips really should remain flexible. High-level fighters have one-third more range of motion in their hips than people who strength train but do not stretch (Keating et al., 2011, *Journal of Strength and Conditioning Research*, 25:S50-1). If you want to keep your range of motion, you need to stretch.

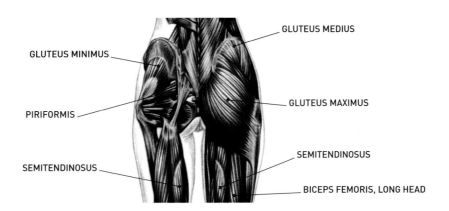

GLUTEUS MEDIUS

GLUTEUS MINIMUS

PIRIFORMIS

GLUTEUS MAXIMUS

SEMITENDINOSUS

SEMITENDINOSUS

BICEPS FEMORIS, LONG HEAD

## HIP ROTATOR STRETCH

*This is a stretch for the piriformis as well as the buttocks. Even though the piriformis is an extremely important muscle, it is often neglected.*

**WHY FIGHTERS SHOULD DO IT**

★ To be able to lift your leg very high when your knee is facing the outside and your foot is facing the inside

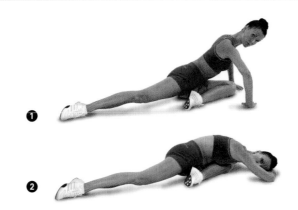

**Lie on the floor and bend one leg in front of you while the other is straight out behind you ❶. Lean your torso forward and rest your hands and forearms on the floor ❷. Hold this position for 20 to 30 seconds before switching to the other leg.**

## HELPFUL HINTS

If you want to make the stretch more intense, lean your torso farther forward.

## VARIATIONS

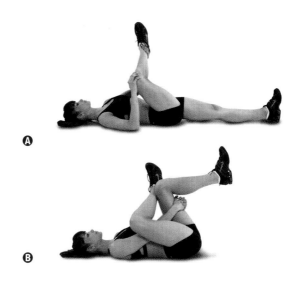

Ⓐ Lie on your back. Put your left leg on the floor and straight out away from your body. Bend your right leg and gently pull your right knee toward your head with your right hand (if necessary). Grab your right ankle with your left hand and bring it toward your head as well.

Ⓑ For an even better stretch, use your left knee to push your right ankle toward your head.

## NOTES

It is very important that you maintain equal flexibility on both sides of your body. Indeed, it is rare for both hips to be equally flexible. Rigid hip rotators drill into the lower back region, making it more prone to injuries.

## ADVANTAGES

This stretch position is identical to the one used in ground fighting.

## DISADVANTAGES

Stretching is not the most exciting form of exercise, but if you want to dominate in a fight, you must perform stretches.

## ⚠ RISKS

When you use the floor or your other leg to do this stretch, it is easy to overstretch the piriformis because it is a very fragile muscle.

# LIFTS AND THROWS

To be able to lift an opponent for a takedown or pick him up for a slam, you absolutely must have powerful muscles in your lower back. Your arms and latissimus dorsi play important roles in pulling an opponent toward you. The best exercises for achieving these goals are deadlifts and weighted pulling exercises.

Since picking up an opponent or flipping him often happens on the ground, variations done on your knees are very important.

## CONVENTIONAL DEADLIFT

*This is a compound exercise for the lumbar muscles, latissimus dorsi, forearms, buttocks, and thighs.*

### WHY FIGHTERS SHOULD DO IT

★ This exercise will give you the total-body strength that is critical for lifting or throwing an opponent; however, this exercise is not specifically designed for fighting.

With your feet a little less than shoulder-width apart, bend over and pick up a bar that you have placed on the floor in front of your ankles ❶. Keep your back flat or very slightly arched. Push with your legs and pull with your back in order to stand up ❷. Synchronize the movement of your legs and back as much as possible: You should not push with your legs first and then pull with your back. Once you are standing up ❸, lean forward while bending your legs to return to the starting position.

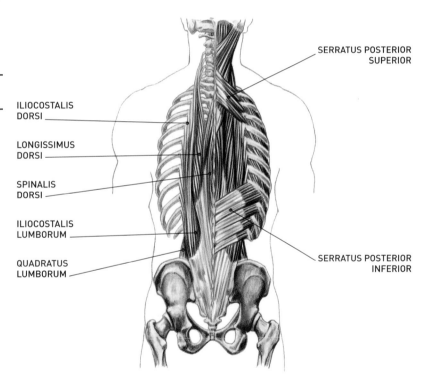

ILIOCOSTALIS DORSI

LONGISSIMUS DORSI

SPINALIS DORSI

ILIOCOSTALIS LUMBORUM

QUADRATUS LUMBORUM

SERRATUS POSTERIOR SUPERIOR

SERRATUS POSTERIOR INFERIOR

**DEEP MUSCLES OF THE BACK USED DURING A DEADLIFT**

### HELPFUL HINTS

When the lower back muscles get tired, it becomes more and more

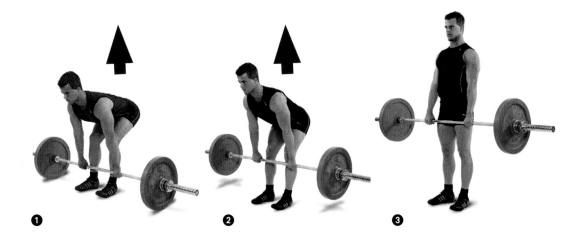

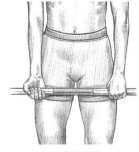

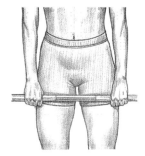

**MIXED GRIP**

**CLASSIC GRIP**

The mixed grip prevents the bar from rolling and allows you to hold much heavier weights.

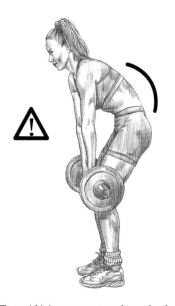

To avoid injury, never round your back during this exercise.

difficult to maintain the slight natural arch of the back. The spine starts to curve, which makes the exercise easier and helps you do a few more repetitions. That is why very few people stop the exercise even though the back is in a horrible position. Continuing the exercise when the lumbar discs are poorly positioned because of fatigue is not a good idea. It is better to stop the exercise the moment you feel your back begin to curve.

## NOTES

Do not do deadlifts rhythmically. Once the bar touches the floor, pause for at least 2 seconds (longer if you are doing midset breaks). In fact, if you start again immediately, you are being aided by the elastic energy that was stored in your muscles as you lowered the bar. When you want to pick up an opponent during a fight, there is no prestretch and therefore no elastic energy built up. Doing deadlifts with a pause in between repetitions is an excellent way to improve your initial strength and acceleration strength.

## VARIATIONS

**Ⓐ** Hand grip is usually mixed, which means that one hand is supinated (thumb toward the outside) and the other is pronated (thumb toward the inside). This grip helps you hold the bar, but the biceps of the supinated hand is extremely vulnerable to tears. Keeping both hands pronated protects the biceps but makes it harder to hold the bar. The classic (pronated) grip is less risky and is the one we recommend you use.

**Ⓑ** You can vary the width of your legs. Choose the width of the stance you use most often during a fight.

**Ⓒ** Instead of using a long bar, you can use two dumbbells. Though it has advantages, this variation shifts your center of gravity too far backward. When you lift an opponent, he is always in front of you, just like the weight bar.

**Ⓓ** Instead of picking the bar up off of the floor, you can place it on a bench or inside a squat rack. This reduces the range of motion and allows you to lift heavier weights while decreasing the risk of a lower back injury. If you only lift your opponents during fights, then this standing variation is the best for you. However, if you do a lot of hand-to-hand fighting on the ground, then the full version is best for your fighting style.

**Ⓔ** The kneeling deadlift is a variation specifically for ground fighting. It prepares you to move or flip an opponent who is on the ground when you are on your knees in front of him. In this position, grab one or two dumbbells from in front of you as you lean your torso forward. Pull your torso back up before lowering to set the weights on the floor. Between repetitions, do not forget to pause for 1 second. To avoid discomfort in the knees, fold a towel or mat and place it under your knees.

## ADVANTAGES

This is the most complete strength training exercise. It works all your muscles in a short time.

## DISADVANTAGES

Because of the sheer number of muscles involved in this exercise, it is exhausting.

 **⚠ WARNING!**

Be sure to warm up your abdominal, oblique, and back muscles well to better support your lower back.

**⚠ RISKS**

This exercise works the spine intensely. There is a serious risk of compressing your intervertebral discs, even with proper positioning. At the end of the workout, you should stretch for a long time at the pull-up bar (see page 50).

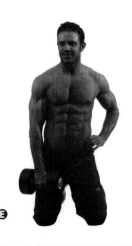

**Ⓔ**

*This is a compound exercise for the hamstrings, buttocks, lumbar region, and back.*

### WHY FIGHTERS SHOULD DO IT

★ This exercise is specifically for ground fighting (see the box on the next page).

**With your feet close together and using a pronated grip, bend forward to pick the bar up off the floor ❶. Keep your back flat and very slightly arched backward. Your legs should be almost straight. Use your hamstrings to stand up as you tightly squeeze your buttocks. Once you are standing up, bend forward again to return to the starting position.**

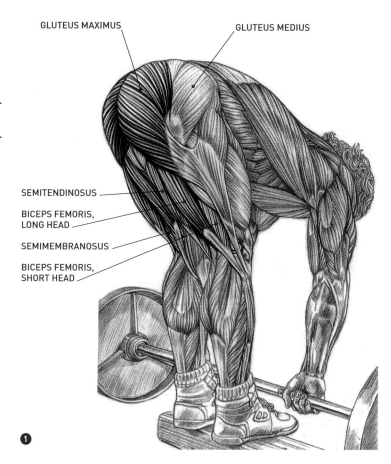

GLUTEUS MAXIMUS

GLUTEUS MEDIUS

SEMITENDINOSUS

BICEPS FEMORIS, LONG HEAD

SEMIMEMBRANOSUS

BICEPS FEMORIS, SHORT HEAD

❶

### HELPFUL HINTS

The farther you lean forward, the more difficult it becomes to maintain the slight natural arch of the back. Your spine will start to curve. In this case, reduce the range of motion by not lowering the bar as far down so that you can always keep your back straight.

To increase the intensity, stand on a board or box so that the feet are higher than the bar on the ground.

### ADVANTAGES

This exercise provides an intense stretch for the hamstrings, so it can cause serious muscle aches.

### DISADVANTAGES

This is a dangerous exercise. When the lumbar muscles grow tired, the spine tends to curve. The trap here is that curving the back gives you a greater range of motion and strength, which is very tempting but also extremely risky.

### ⚠ RISKS

The spine is heavily compressed in this exercise, even if you do it with perfect form.

## DIFFERENCES BETWEEN THE STRAIGHT-LEG DEADLIFT AND THE CONVENTIONAL DEADLIFT

The straight-leg deadlift has the following characteristics:

→ It is a variation of the conventional deadlift and is specifically for ground fighting. In fact, when you are standing up and you lean forward to pick up or flip an opponent who is on the ground, you are in the straight-leg deadlift position.

→ It puts the lower back into an even more precarious position because it requires you to lean farther forward than a conventional deadlift.

→ It recruits the hamstrings more and the quadriceps less than a conventional deadlift.

### NOTES

The straight-leg deadlift more closely matches ground fighting than it does fighting while standing upright. This will make it easy for you to choose between the two versions. In fact, we recommend that you not do both forms of deadlifts during the same workout so that you will not overwork your lower back.

## DUMBBELL CLEAN

*This is a compound exercise for the lumbar region, latissimus dorsi, arms, buttocks, thighs, and calves. The shoulders also work very hard in the version where you lift your arms above your head. Weightlifters call that variation a clean and press.*

### WHY FIGHTERS SHOULD DO IT

★ This is the most complete exercise that exists because all the muscles in the body participate.

★ Even though this exercise is not specifically for fighting, the lifting part gives beginners the critical total-body strength required for dominating with strength in hand-to-hand fighting.

**Bend over so you can pick up two dumbbells that are next to your feet. Keep your back flat or arched very slightly ❶. Use a natural hand grip—semipronated (thumbs forward and turned slightly toward each other) is ideal.**

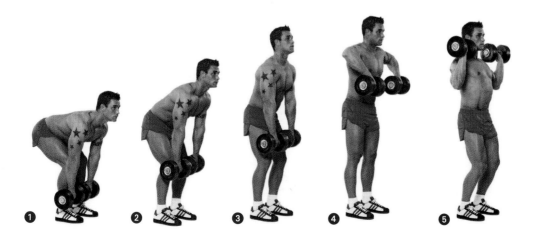

Push with your legs and pull with your back to stand up ❷ ❸. Synchronize your leg and back movements as much as possible. Once you are almost standing up, use your momentum to bend your arms (hands almost pronated) ❹ and bring the weights to shoulder level ❺. From there, lower the weights and lean forward as you bend your legs to return to the starting position.

### HELPFUL HINTS

Be sure to warm up very well before using heavy weights. Your warm-up should not only prepare your muscles but also condition you for the technical execution of the exercise.

### NOTES

Keep your head very straight and gaze slightly upward. Most important, avoid looking left or right because that could make you lose your balance and result in a back injury.

### VARIATIONS

❹ For a more complete exercise that recruits the shoulders and triceps, you can straighten your arms above your head to perform the clean using full range of motion. This is a more complex variation

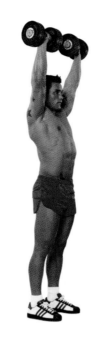

Ⓐ

and is not recommended for beginners who have less than three months of experience in strength training.

❸ Weightlifters often use a long bar in this exercise. However, this variation provides rigidity and symmetry in the exercise that you will never experience in a fight.

### ADVANTAGES

The clean works all the major muscle groups in a short time. Not only does it work the muscles, it also helps improve motor coordination. Since you can do the exercise explosively, it creates a lot of power. When you do it in long sets, it is also excellent for increasing muscular endurance.

### DISADVANTAGES

This is a very technical exercise. It requires a certain amount of time to learn how to do it and to gain muscle mastery.

### ⚠ RISKS

The explosiveness of this exercise can be dangerous. You must begin this exercise with extreme caution. Do not start out right away with heavy weights.

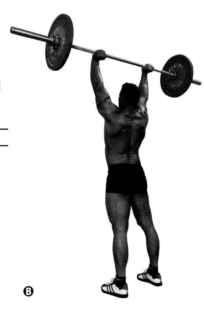

Ⓑ

*This is a compound exercise that focuses on all the back muscles as well as the biceps, forearms, and thighs.*

### WHY FIGHTERS SHOULD DO IT

★ This exercise is similar to the position in hand-to-hand fighting where you stand up and lean forward in order to pick up or flip over an opponent who is on the ground.

★ This exercise will also give you the necessary strength to knock an opponent off balance by pulling him toward you when you are both standing up during a fight.

**Lean forward so that your torso forms a 90- to 145-degree angle to the floor. Grab two dumbbells or kettlebells with a neutral grip (thumbs forward) ❶. Pull with your arms and bring your elbows up as high as possible ❷. Squeeze your shoulder blades together before you lower the weights.**

### HELPFUL HINTS

As a general rule, you should pull the dumbbells up to your navel. Some people like to bring the weights a little higher

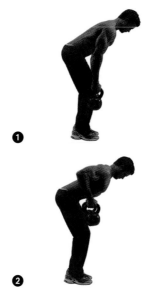

toward the chest and others a little lower, near the thighs. In the same way, for hand positions, some people prefer to have the thumbs slightly turned in and others like them slightly turned out. Choose the position that most closely matches what you encounter in your fighting discipline.

### NOTES

Keep your head high, especially during the contraction phase of the exercise. Do not turn your head from left to right.

### VARIATION

A kneeling variation is specifically for ground fighting. It involves moving or lifting an opponent who is lying on

the ground while you are on your knees and in side control. In this position, lean forward and grab one or two dumbbells from in front of you to do the rowing exercise. Between each repetition, let go of the dumbbell for 1 second before starting the exercise again.

When you are on your knees, the difficulty lies in keeping your balance by anchoring your tibia to the floor through a powerful contraction of the quadriceps. To prevent knee discomfort, fold up a towel or a mat and place it on the floor so you can kneel on it.

### ADVANTAGES

Rowing works all of the muscles used for pulling in a coordinated manner, no matter what position you are in (standing or kneeling).

### DISADVANTAGES

The forward leaning position is very hard on the spine.

### ⚠ RISKS

Even though leaning forward 145 degrees is less risky than 90 degrees, rowing is still risky for the back, especially when you are using heavy weights.

## JUST BECAUSE SOMETHING IS POPULAR DOES NOT MEAN IT WORKS

Here is very popular exercise among fighters: Lift yourself with your arms and back while your body is more or less parallel to the floor as you look at the ceiling. However, this exercise does not correspond to any fighting movement, because you never pull an opponent when your lower back and thighs are relaxed. When you pull with your arms or your back, you need your lower back muscles to transmit strength to your thighs perfectly so that your body is anchored to the floor. To compensate for this weakness in the exercise, you would have to do an isolation exercise to strengthen your sacrolumbar muscles and another isolation exercise for your thighs.

But if you replace this exercise with rowing while leaning forward, you will work your arms, back, legs, and lower back all at the same time. Of course, this exercise is harder, because it recruits the entire body.

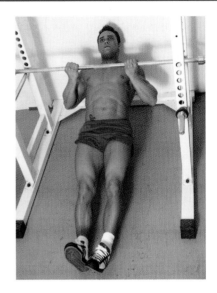

However, it is also more productive and takes less time to do than if you did several isolation exercises that are not as important for a fighter.

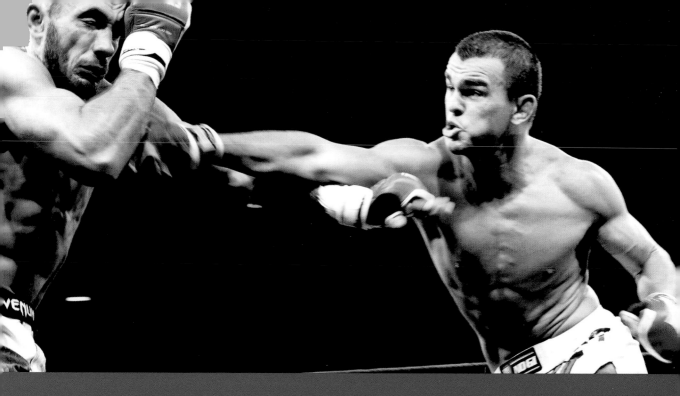

BY NOW WE HOPE YOU UNDERSTAND THAT YOU MUST CUSTOMIZE YOUR STRENGTH TRAINING PROGRAM TO MEET THE REQUIREMENTS OF YOUR FIGHTING DISCIPLINE, NOT ADJUST YOUR TRAINING TO MEET THE CONSTRAINTS OF WHATEVER STRENGTH TRAINING PROGRAM YOU ARE FOLLOWING. WE HAVE INCLUDED A GREAT DEAL OF ADVICE IN ALL THE EXERCISES. EXAMPLES OF OPTIMAL PROGRAMS ARE PROVIDED FOR YOU IN PART 3 OF THIS BOOK. THESE WILL HELP YOU WORK THE NECESSARY MUSCLE GROUPS WITHOUT TAKING TIME AWAY FROM YOUR FIGHT TRAINING.

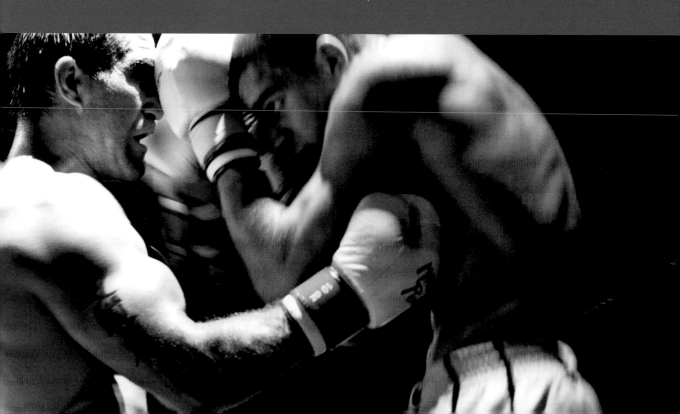

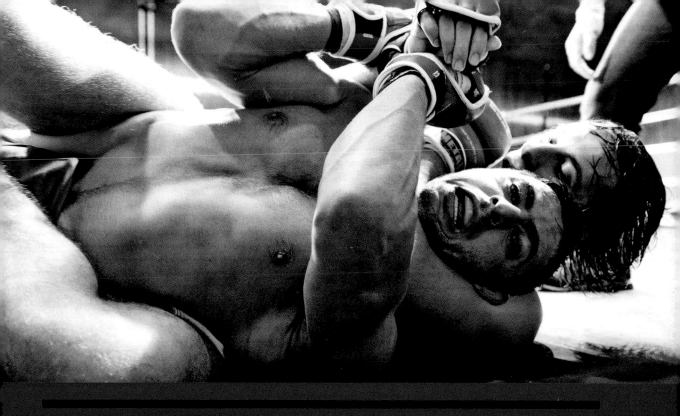

# TRAINING PROGRAMS

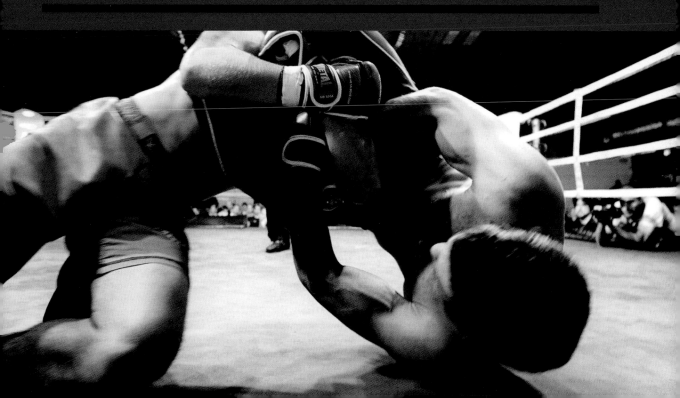

If you have never done strength training, it is important to start with a total-body strengthening program so you can quickly increase your muscle strength. You should start with general strength training techniques so you can learn to perform basic exercises properly, position your back correctly, and breathe properly.

These programs are not customized for fighting, but they are easier than specific strength training programs. You have to learn to walk before you can run; it will keep you from stumbling! Once you have mastered basic technique, choose one of the customized fighting programs so you can develop strength, speed, power, and endurance.

## PROGRAM FOR GAINING FAMILIARITY WITH STRENGTH TRAINING

Do this program 1 or 2 times each week for 1 month.

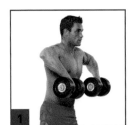
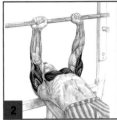
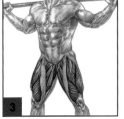
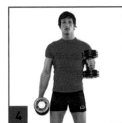

**1** **DUMBBELL CLEAN**     p. 121

2 sets of 12 to 8 repetitions

**2** **NARROW-GRIP BENCH PRESS**     p. 81

3 sets of 10 to 6 repetitions

**3** **PARTIAL SQUAT**     p. 90

3 sets of 12 to 8 repetitions

**4** **HAMMER CURL**     p. 104

2 sets of 20 to 12 repetitions

## PROGRAM FOR INCREASING VOLUME OF WORK

Begin this program once you feel comfortable with the beginning program. Do 2 workouts each week.

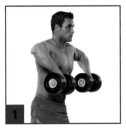
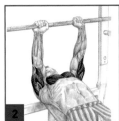

**1** **DUMBBELL CLEAN**     p. 121

2 sets of 10 to 4 repetitions

**2** **NARROW-GRIP BENCH PRESS**     p. 81

3 sets of 8 to 4 repetitions

**PARTIAL SQUAT** p. 90

3 sets of 10 to 6 repetitions

**SIT-UP** p. 70

2 sets of 20 to 12 repetitions

**ROW** p. 123

2 sets of 12 to 8 repetitions

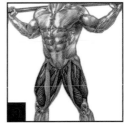
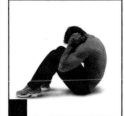
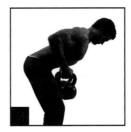
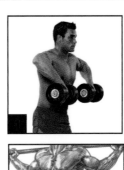

## ADVANCED BEGINNER PROGRAM

After 2 to 3 months, move on to this advanced beginner program. Do at least 2 workouts each week.

**DUMBBELL CLEAN** p. 121

3 sets of 10 to 4 repetitions

**NARROW-GRIP
BENCH PRESS** p.81

3 sets of 8 to 4 repetitions

**PARTIAL SQUAT** p. 90

3 sets of 10 to 6 repetitions

**SIT-UP** p. 70

2 sets of 20 to 12 repetitions

**ROW** p. 123

2 sets of 12 to 8 repetitions

**POWER TRICEPS PUSH-DOWN** p. 101

2 sets of 12 to 8 repetitions

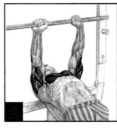
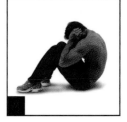
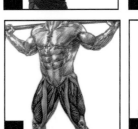
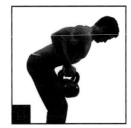
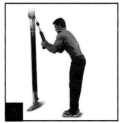

After several months of beginner training, select a program that is designed for fighting. Ideally, you should do at least 1 specialized program per week plus 1 circuit training workout on another day (see sections starting on page 135).

## BASIC SPECIALIZED PROGRAM

**1 PUNCH WITH A PULLEY**     p. 83

3 sets of 8 to 4 repetitions

**2 STRAIGHT-LEG DEADLIFT**     p. 120

3 sets of 10 to 6 repetitions

**3 MEDICINE BALL THROW**     p. 85

3 sets of 20 repetitions

**4 PARTIAL SQUAT**     p. 90

3 sets of 10 to 6 repetitions

**5 WRIST EXTENSION**     p. 87

2 sets of 20 to 12 repetitions

**6 TWISTING CRUNCH**     p. 74

2 sets of 12 to 8 repetitions

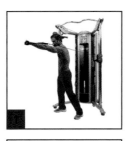
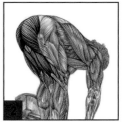
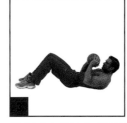
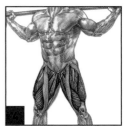
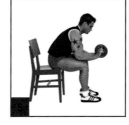
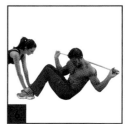
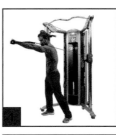

## ADVANCED SPECIALIZED PROGRAM

**1 PUNCH WITH A PULLEY**     p. 83

3 sets of 8 to 4 repetitions

**2 STRAIGHT-LEG DEADLIFT**     p. 120

2 sets of 10 to 6 repetitions

**3 MEDICINE BALL THROW**     p. 85

3 sets of 20 repetitions

**4 PARTIAL SQUAT**     p. 90

2 sets of 10 to 6 repetitions

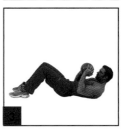
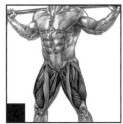
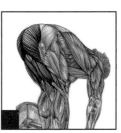

**TWISTING CRUNCH** p. 74

2 sets of 12 to 8 repetitions

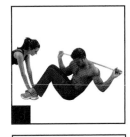

**ROW** p. 123

2 sets of 12 to 8 repetitions

**WRIST EXTENSION** p. 87

2 sets of 20 to 12 repetitions

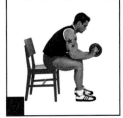
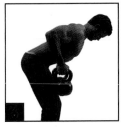

**HANG FROM PULL-UP BAR** p. 102

2 sets of 30 to 20 repetitions

**ISOMETRIC ADDUCTION** p. 106

1 set of 5 to 3 repetitions,
each held for at least 30 seconds

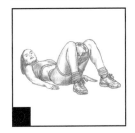
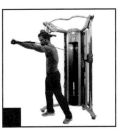

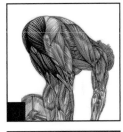

## HIGHLY ADVANCED SPECIALIZED PROGRAM

**PUNCH WITH A PULLEY** p. 83

2 sets of 8 to 4 repetitions

**STANDING LEG LIFT** p. 96

2 sets of 10 to 6 repetitions

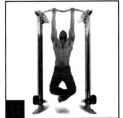

**STRAIGHT-LEG DEADLIFT** p. 120

2 sets of 10 to 6 repetitions

**MEDICINE BALL THROW** p. 85

2 sets of 20 repetitions

**PARTIAL SQUAT** p. 90

2 sets of 10 to 6 repetitions

**TWISTING CRUNCH** p. 74

2 sets of 12 to 8 repetitions

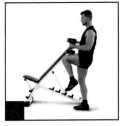
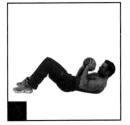

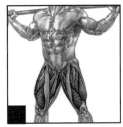
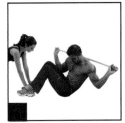

### ROW                                           p. 123

2 sets of 12 to 8 repetitions

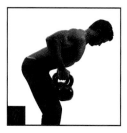

### ISOMETRIC ADDUCTION                            p. 106

1 set of 6 to 3 repetitions,
each held for at least 30 seconds

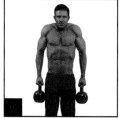
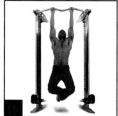

### SHRUG                                          p. 66

2 sets of 10 to 6 repetitions

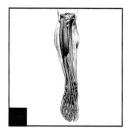

### HANG FROM PULL-UP BAR                          p. 102

2 sets of 30 to 20 repetitions

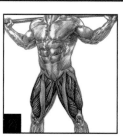

### REVERSE CALF RAISE                             p. 111

1 set of 6 to 4 repetitions,
each held for at least 30 seconds

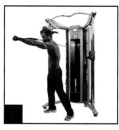

To focus more on improving certain strikes, choose an even more specialized strengthening program. Ideally, you should do at least 2 specialized workouts each week plus 1 circuit training workout on another day (see sections starting on page 137).

## BOXING PROGRAM

### PUNCH WITH A PULLEY                            p. 83

5 sets of 12 to 8 repetitions

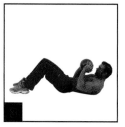
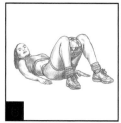

### PARTIAL SQUAT                                  p. 90

3 sets of 10 to 6 repetitions

### MEDICINE BALL THROW                            p. 85

3 sets of 15 repetitions

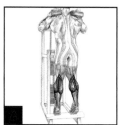

### STANDING CALF RAISE                           p. 92

3 sets of 20 to 10 repetitions

**■ WRIST EXTENSION IN NONSTOP SUPERSET WITH**
**■ WRIST CURL** p. 88 and p. 89

3 supersets of 20 to 15 repetitions

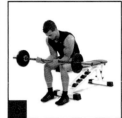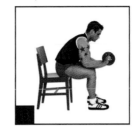

## KICKING PROGRAM

**■ STANDING LEG LIFT** p. 96

4 sets of 8 to 4 repetitions

**■ PARTIAL SQUAT** p. 90

3 sets of 10 to 6 repetitions

**■ LEG LIFT ON PULL-UP BAR** p. 98

3 sets of 20 to 10 repetitions

**■ KNEE STRIKE ON ALL FOURS** p. 99

4 sets of 10 to 6 repetitions

**■ SIT-UP** p. 70

3 sets of 25 to 12 repetitions

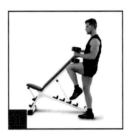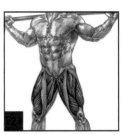

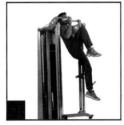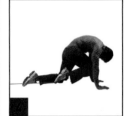

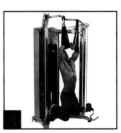

## GROUND FIGHTING PROGRAM

**■ LEG PRESS USING FULL RANGE OF MOTION** p. 108

3 sets of 10 to 6 repetitions

**■ HANG FROM STRAPS** p. 105

1 set of 6 to 3 repetitions,
each held for at least 30 seconds

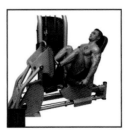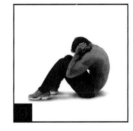

**ISOMETRIC ADDUCTION**     p. 106

1 set of 6 to 3 repetitions,
each held for at least 30 seconds

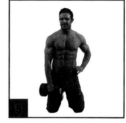

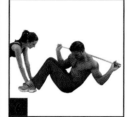

**REVERSE CALF RAISE**     p. 111

1 set of 6 to 3 repetitions,
each held for at least 30 seconds

**KNEELING DEADLIFT**     p. 119

3 sets of 20 to 12 repetitions

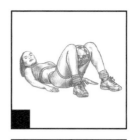

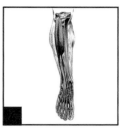

**TWISTING CRUNCH**     p. 74

3 sets of 25 to 12 repetitions

# HAND-TO-HAND FIGHTING PROGRAM

**PARTIAL SQUAT**     p. 90

4 sets of 10 to 6 repetitions

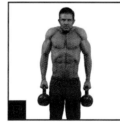

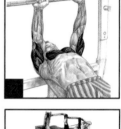

**NARROW-GRIP
BENCH PRESS**     p. 81

4 sets of 10 to 6 repetitions

**KNEELING DEADLIFT**     p. 119

3 sets of 20 to 12 repetitions

**HANG FROM STRAPS**     p. 105

1 set of 6 to 3 repetitions,
each held for at least 30 seconds

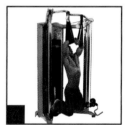

**SHRUG**     p. 66

3 sets of 8 to 6 repetitions

**STANDING CALF RAISE**     p. 92

3 sets of 20 to 10 repetitions

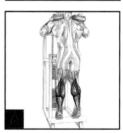

To improve your cardiorespiratory fitness, choose a circuit training program. Introduce circuits progressively after 1 to 2 months of basic strength training.

## BEGINNER BASIC CIRCUIT

Do 2 or 3 circuits of 15 to 20 repetitions each with minimal rest time between sets. Do this workout at least 1 time per week.

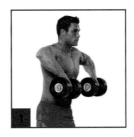
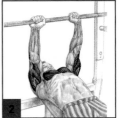

**1 DUMBBELL CLEAN**     p. 121

15 to 20 repetitions

**2 NARROW-GRIP BENCH PRESS**     p. 81

15 to 20 repetitions

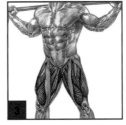
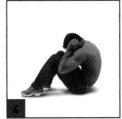

**3 PARTIAL SQUAT**     p. 90

15 to 20 repetitions

**4 SIT-UP**     p. 70

15 to 20 repetitions

## INTERMEDIATE BASIC CIRCUIT

Do 3 or 4 circuits of 15 to 20 repetitions each with minimal rest time between exercises. Do this workout at least 1 time per week.

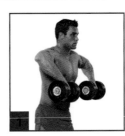
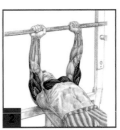

**1 DUMBBELL CLEAN**     p. 121

15 to 20 repetitions

**2 NARROW-GRIP BENCH PRESS**     p. 81

15 to 20 repetitions

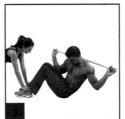
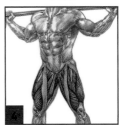

**3 TWISTING CRUNCH**     p. 74

15 to 20 repetitions

**4 PARTIAL SQUAT**     p. 90

15 to 20 repetitions

**▣ SIT-UP**     p. 70

15 to 20 repetitions

> **Note:** Do a few circuits while wearing a mouth guard because it restricts your breathing somewhat, especially if you are not used to wearing one.

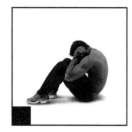

# ADVANCED BASIC CIRCUIT

Do 3 or 4 circuits of 15 to 20 repetitions each with no rest time between exercises. Do this workout at least 2 times each week.

**▣ DUMBBELL CLEAN**     p. 121

15 to 20 repetitions

**▣ NARROW-GRIP BENCH PRESS**     p. 81

15 to 20 repetitions

**▣ PARTIAL SQUAT**     p. 90

15 to 20 repetitions

**▣ SIT-UP**     p. 70

15 to 20 repetitions

**▣ ROW**     p. 123

15 to 20 repetitions

**▣ LYING RIB CAGE EXPANSION**     p. 114

At least 50 repetitions

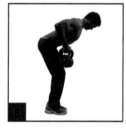
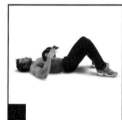
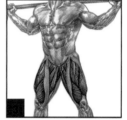
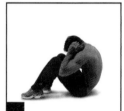
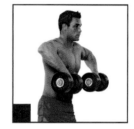
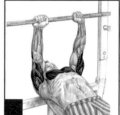

To increase both your endurance and the effectiveness of certain strikes, choose a more customized circuit.

## BOXING CIRCUIT

Do 3 to 5 circuits of 15 to 20 repetitions with no rest time between exercises. Do this workout at least 1 time each week.

**PUNCH WITH A PULLEY**     p. 83

15 to 20 repetitions

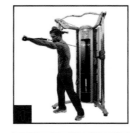 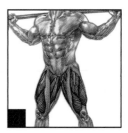

**PARTIAL SQUAT**     p. 90

15 to 20 repetitions

**MEDICINE BALL THROW**     p. 85

15 to 20 repetitions

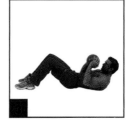 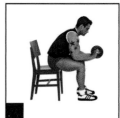

**WRIST EXTENSION**     p. 87

15 to 20 repetitions

**LYING RIB CAGE EXPANSION**     p. 114

At least 50 repetitions

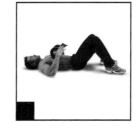

## KICKING CIRCUIT

Do 3 to 5 circuits of 15 to 20 repetitions each with no rest time between exercises. Do this workout at least 1 time each week.

**STANDING LEG LIFT**     p. 96

15 to 20 repetitions

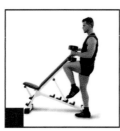 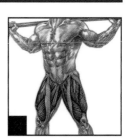

**PARTIAL SQUAT**     p. 90

15 to 20 repetitions

**SIT-UP**     p. 70

15 to 20 repetitions

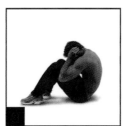 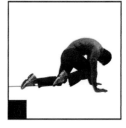

**KNEE STRIKE ON ALL FOURS**     p. 99

15 to 20 repetitions

**LYING RIB CAGE EXPANSION**      p. 114

At least 50 repetitions

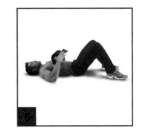

---

# GROUND FIGHTING CIRCUIT

Do 3 or 4 circuits of 15 to 20 repetitions with no rest time between exercises. Do this workout at least 1 time each week.

**LEG PRESS USING FULL RANGE OF MOTION**      p. 108

15 to 20 repetitions

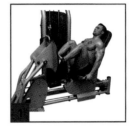
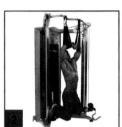

**HANG FROM STRAPS**      p. 105

15 to 20 repetitions

**ISOMETRIC ADDUCTION**      p. 106

3 repetitions, each held for at least 30 seconds

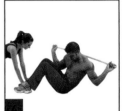

**TWISTING CRUNCH**      p. 74

15 to 20 repetitions

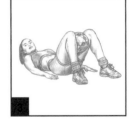
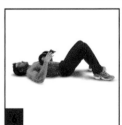

**KNEELING DEADLIFT**      p. 119

15 to 20 repetitions

**LYING RIB CAGE EXPANSION**      p.114

At least 50 repetitions

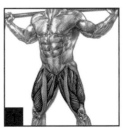
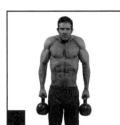

---

# HAND-TO-HAND FIGHTING CIRCUIT

Do 3 or 4 circuits of 12 to 15 repetitions with no rest time between exercises. Do this workout at least 1 time each week.

**PARTIAL SQUAT**      p. 90

12 to 15 repetitions

**SHRUG**      p. 66

12 to 15 repetitions

**HANG FROM STRAPS**                    p. 105

3 repetitions, each held for at least 30 seconds

**NARROW-GRIP
BENCH PRESS**                           p. 81

12 to 15 repetitions

**KNEELING DEADLIFT**                   p. 119

12 to 15 repetitions

**LYING RIB CAGE EXPANSION**           p. 114

At least 50 repetitions

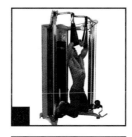
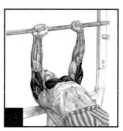
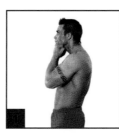
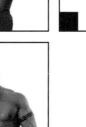

# SPECIALIZED CIRCUITS AT HOME

The neck and abdominal wall are two muscle groups that you can strengthen in an isolated manner at home with little equipment required. This will save you time at the gym.

## SPECIALIZED CIRCUITS FOR PROTECTING THE NECK

Do 3 to 5 circuits of 20 to 30 repetitions with no rest time between exercises. Do this workout 2 or 3 times each week.

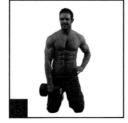

**NECK FLEXION**                        p. 60

20 to 30 repetitions

**NECK EXTENSION**                      p. 61

20 to 30 repetitions

**LATERAL NECK FLEXION**               p. 63

20 to 30 repetitions

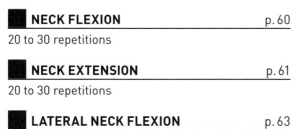

## SPECIALIZED CIRCUIT FOR ABDOMINAL SUPPORT

Do 4 to 6 circuits with no rest time between exercises. Do this workout 2 or 3 times each week.

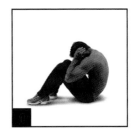 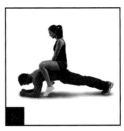

■ **SIT-UP** p. 70

50 to 30 repetitions

■ **PLANK** p. 78

At least 30 seconds

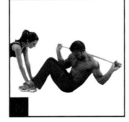 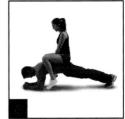

■ **TWISTING CRUNCH** p. 74

30 to 15 repetitions per side

■ **PLANK** p. 78

At least 30 seconds

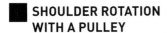

# CIRCUITS FOR INJURY PREVENTION

Even slight joint pain will negatively affect your performance. Targeted strength training programs can help prevent the most common injuries encountered in fighting. Here, your goal is to consolidate the weak links in your most exposed joints.

## PREVENTING SHOULDER PAIN

*Since combat sports require an enormous amount of movement in the shoulders, they can cause pain in your deltoids. To prevent this trauma, you need to maintain stability in your joints by strengthening the supporting muscles. This includes the back of the shoulder, infraspinatus, and lower trapezius (see page 65).*

Do 3 to 5 circuits of 15 to 25 repetitions with no rest time between exercises at least 2 times each week. Include this circuit as a warm-up at the beginning of your strength training or fight workouts.

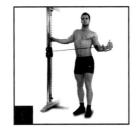 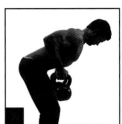

■ **SHOULDER ROTATION WITH A PULLEY** p. 85

15 to 25 repetitions

■ **ROW** p. 123

15 to 25 repetitions

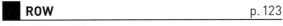

## PREVENTING LOWER BACK PAIN

*The lower back is worked intensely during a fight. To prevent lower back pain, you should strengthen the muscles that support the spine. This includes the abdominal muscles (especially the lower part), obliques, and back muscles.*

Do 2 to 4 circuits of 15 to 25 repetitions with minimal rest time between exercises at least 1 time each week. Include this circuit at the end of your strength training or fight workouts.

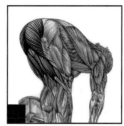
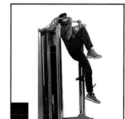

**1 STRAIGHT-LEG DEADLIFT** p. 120

15 to 25 repetitions

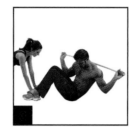

**2 LEG LIFT ON PULL-UP BAR** p. 98

15 to 25 repetitions

**3 TWISTING CRUNCH** p. 74

15 to 25 repetitions

## PREVENTING NECK PAIN

*As soon as there is any contact, the neck suffers intense abuse. To protect it, you should strengthen the muscles that stabilize the neck as well as upper trapezius muscles.*

Do this circuit at least 2 times each week with no rest time between exercises. Do it at the end of your strength training or fight workouts.

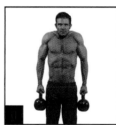
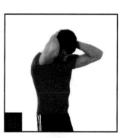

**1 SHRUG** p. 66

8 to 12 repetitions

**2 NECK EXTENSION** p. 61

20 to 30 repetitions

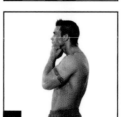
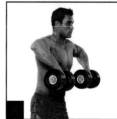

**3 NECK FLEXION** p. 60

20 to 30 repetitions

**4 DUMBBELL CLEAN** p. 121

8 to 12 repetitions

**5 LATERAL NECK FLEXION** p. 63

20 to 30 repetitions

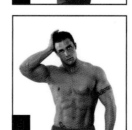

# PREVENTING HIP PAIN

*Abrupt rotations of the hips can easily damage the small muscles that control the direction of the thighs. This means you need to strengthen and stretch these muscles.*

Do 2 or 3 circuits of 20 to 10 repetitions at least 2 times each week. Instead of doing the exercises back to back, take 30 seconds to stretch in between exercises. Include this circuit at the very beginning or the very end of your strength training workouts.

**1 ISOMETRIC ADDUCTION** — p. 106

20 to 10 repetitions,
each held for at least 30 seconds

**2 HIP ROTATOR STRETCH** — p. 115

At least 30 seconds on each side

**3 LYING LEG CURL** — p. 109

20 to 10 repetitions

**4 HIP ROTATOR STRETCH** — p. 115

At least 30 seconds on each side

**5 STRAIGHT-LEG DEADLIFT** — p. 120

20 to 10 repetitions

**6 HIP ROTATOR STRETCH** — p. 115

At least 30 seconds on each side

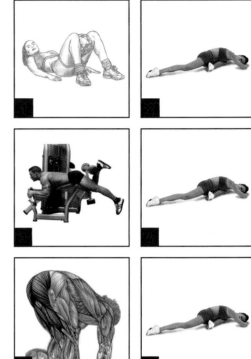

## PREVENTING KNEE PAIN AND HAMSTRING TEARS

*Knee problems are very common in combat sports. They often occur because of a strength imbalance between the hamstrings and quadriceps. Strength training programs generally focus on the quadriceps and neglect the hamstrings, even though the hamstrings are more important in fighting.*

*This puts the knee joint in a precarious position, because the tension is not balanced. A strength training program should balance out that tension. In addition, strengthening the hamstrings will also help prevent hamstring tears.*

Do 2 or 3 circuits of 10 to 25 repetitions at least 2 times each week. Include this circuit as a warm-up at the very beginning of your workout.

**1 CONVENTIONAL DEADLIFT** p. 117

10 to 25 repetitions

**2 HIP ROTATOR STRETCH** p. 115

At least 30 seconds on each side

**3 LEG PRESS USING FULL RANGE OF MOTION** p. 108

10 to 25 repetitions

**4 HIP ROTATOR STRETCH** p. 115

At least 30 seconds on each side

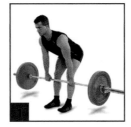
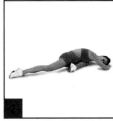
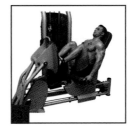
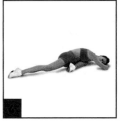

**Library of Congress Cataloging-in-Publication Data**

Delavier, Frédéric.
  [Musculation pour le fight et les sports de combat. English]
  Delavier's mixed martial arts anatomy / Frédéric Delavier, Michael Gundill.
    pages cm
  Includes bibliographical references.
  1. Exercise--Physiological aspects. 2. Human anatomy. 3. Martial arts. I. Gundill, Michael. II. Title. III. Title:
Mixed martial arts anatomy.
  QP301.D33813 2013
  612'.044--dc23
                              2013012265

ISBN-10: 1-4504-6359-2 (print)
ISBN-13: 978-1-4504-6359-1 (print)

Original title in French, *Musculation Pour le Fight et les Sports de Combat,* copyright © 2012 by Éditions Vigot, 23,
rue de l'École-de-Médecine, 75006 Paris, France.

English language version, *Delavier's Mixed Martial Arts Anatomy,* copyright © 2013 by Human Kinetics, Inc.

This publication is written and published to provide accurate and authoritative information relevant to the subject
matter presented. It is published and sold with the understanding that the author and publisher are not engaged in
rendering legal, medical, or other professional services by reason of their authorship or publication of this work. If
medical or other expert assistance is required, the services of a competent professional person should be sought.

This book is a revised edition of *Musculation Pour le Fight et les Sports de Combat,* published in 2012 by Éditions
Vigot.

Photography: © All rights reserved, except for pages 6, 11, 55, 125, 127: © Yann Levy; Illustrations: © All illustrations
by Frédéric Delavier; Graphics conception and direction: Claire Guigal; Editing: Sophie Lilienfeld; Photoengraving:
IGS

Human Kinetics books are available at special discounts for bulk purchase. Special editions or book excerpts can
also be created to specification. For details, contact the Special Sales Manager at Human Kinetics.

Printed in France    10 9 8 7 6 5 4 3 2 1

**Human Kinetics**
Website: www.HumanKinetics.com

*United States:* Human Kinetics
P.O. Box 5076
Champaign, IL 61825-5076
800-747-4457
e-mail: humank@hkusa.com

*Canada:* Human Kinetics
475 Devonshire Road Unit 100
Windsor, ON N8Y 2L5
800-465-7301 (in Canada only)
e-mail: info@hkcanada.com

*Europe:* Human Kinetics
107 Bradford Road
Stanningley
Leeds LS28 6AT, United Kingdom
+44 (0) 113 255 5665
e-mail: hk@hkeurope.com

*Australia:* Human Kinetics
57A Price Avenue
Lower Mitcham, South Australia 5062
08 8372 0999
e-mail: info@hkaustralia.com

*New Zealand:* Human Kinetics
P.O. Box 80
Torrens Park, South Australia 5062
0800 222 062
e-mail: info@hknewzealand.com

E6035